I0783186

My Peace of Health

© 2024 - My Peace of Health, LLC

My Peace of Health

A Faith-Based Guide to Peaceful Living

by Candice Leanos

© 2024 - My Peace of Health, LLC

© 2024 - My Peace of Health, LLC

Copyright © 2024 Candice Leanos

All rights reserved. No part of this publication may be reproduced, distributed, or transmitted in any form or by any means, including photocopying, recording, or other electronic or mechanical methods, without the prior written permission of the author, except in the case of brief quotations embodied in critical reviews and certain other noncommercial uses permitted by copyright law.

For permissions requests, write to the author at the address below:

My Peace of Health LLC

Mypeaceofhealth@gmail.com

www.mypeaceofhealth.com

Printed in United States of America

First Printing: May, 2024

© 2024 - My Peace of Health, LLC

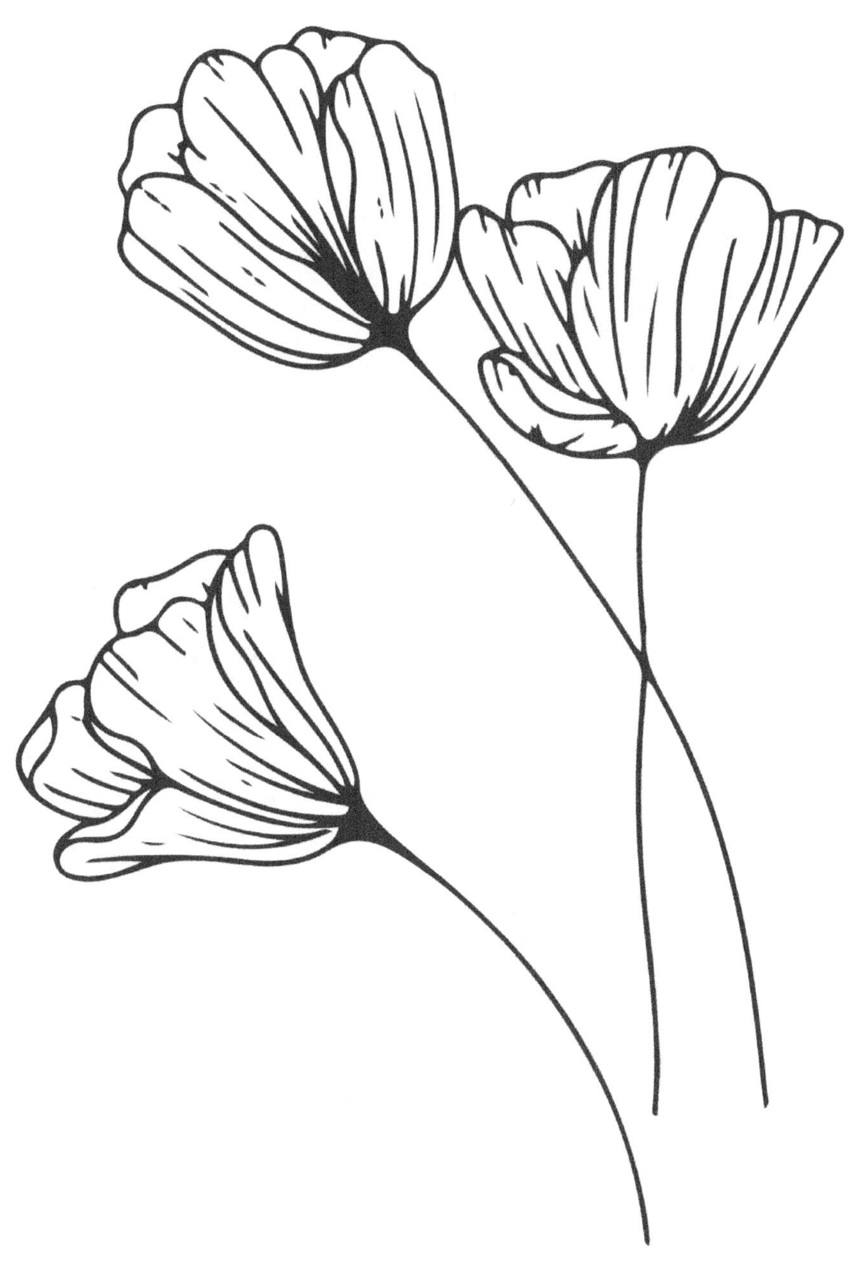

© 2024 - My Peace of Health, LLC

© 2024 - My Peace of Health, LLC

To my beloved husband Simon, and our precious children,

Patricia, **E**lijah, **A**rmon, **C**aliana, and **E**than,

Your love and presence bring PEACE to my life every day. Thank you for being my constant source of joy, strength, and inspiration. Together, we navigate life's journey with faith, hope, and endless love.

With all my heart,

Mom

© 2024 - My Peace of Health, LLC

© 2024 - My Peace of Health, LLC

FOREWORD

Considering the uncertainty and chaos in our world today, it can seem like an impossible task to find peace. It is easy for us to lose focus on what is most important as we navigate the complexities of life.

My Peace of Health offers us a beacon of hope. Through her personal journey of adversity and triumph, Candice Leanos shares a roadmap to faith-based peaceful living. With vulnerability, grace, and wisdom, she shares invaluable insights on self-care, wellness, and holistic practices.

Her authenticity is refreshing as she intertwines personal experiences with practical tips for nurturing our minds, bodies, and spirits. The pages resonate with warmth and encouragement as Candice touches on navigating relationships, dealing with change, and cultivating inner peace.

It has been a privilege and honor for me to witness Candice's transformative journey to healing and wholeness. I have known her since she was a child, and I was a young adult. Although I am a physician and wellness coach, Candice has been an inspiration to me in my quest for peace and health. Her services as my personal fitness coach have benefited me greatly. I'm grateful she has decided to author and share this book so that others may benefit from her experience and expertise.

May this book be your guide as you embark on your transformative journey to healthful living and holistic wellness.

-Karla Montague-Brown, M.D
Founder-CEO of CROWN TO SOLE Wellness, LLC
Author of "**Overcoming Autoimmunity**: One physician's step-by-step journey to victory over her chronic illnesses."

© 2024 - My Peace of Health, LLC

© 2024 - My Peace of Health, LLC

Table of Contents

© 2024 - My Peace of Health, LLC

© 2024 - My Peace of Health, LLC

© 2024 - My Peace of Health, LLC

© 2024 - My Peace of Health, LLC

Hey there!

Welcome to 'My Peace of Health: Faith-based Guide for a Peaceful Life'. My name is Candice. I'm the wife of an incredible hubby Simon and the momma of five kiddos ranging from kindergarten cuties to young adults soaring. I'm a natural-born hard worker who understands that life as a wife and momma can feel chaotic at times..

Being real, I've been through and experienced more than I thought possible, the peaks and valleys of motherhood, to the day-to-day highs and lows of marriage and more. What has survived through it all? My faith and my pursuit of peace.

So, I launched My Peace of Health LLC, a coaching service where I help you on your journey and share a passion for holistic wellness grounded in plant-based nutrition, exercise and spiritual fitness. Let's face it, true peace comes from within—when our bodies, minds and spirits are nourished, revitalized and robust. And we serve a risen king, not a future king—so peace isn't some future hope—it's possible today, right now.

I invite you to join me on that journey towards deeper connection, joy, and resilience in "My Peace of Health", where we will discuss the what, why, and how of 'living well' from a Christian perspective, including practical common sense, beautiful stories, and 'a life hack' or two – how to feel calm and connected even in the midst of chaos and madness. Whether you're in the struggle of mom life, trying to survive the ups and downs of marriage, or simply trying to find more meaning and peace, this book is for you, sis.

So, grab your favorite drink, find a comfy chair and prepare for a wonderful flight toward truth, love and living bright 'cause peace isn't merely something we seek: it's something you breathe every single day. Cheers to our unique journey, to becoming more whole, to becoming more at peace and having more joy in our everyday living – Go in peace, with a smile.

With love and gratitude,
Candice Leanos

© 2024 - My Peace of Health, LLC

© 2024 - My Peace of Health, LLC

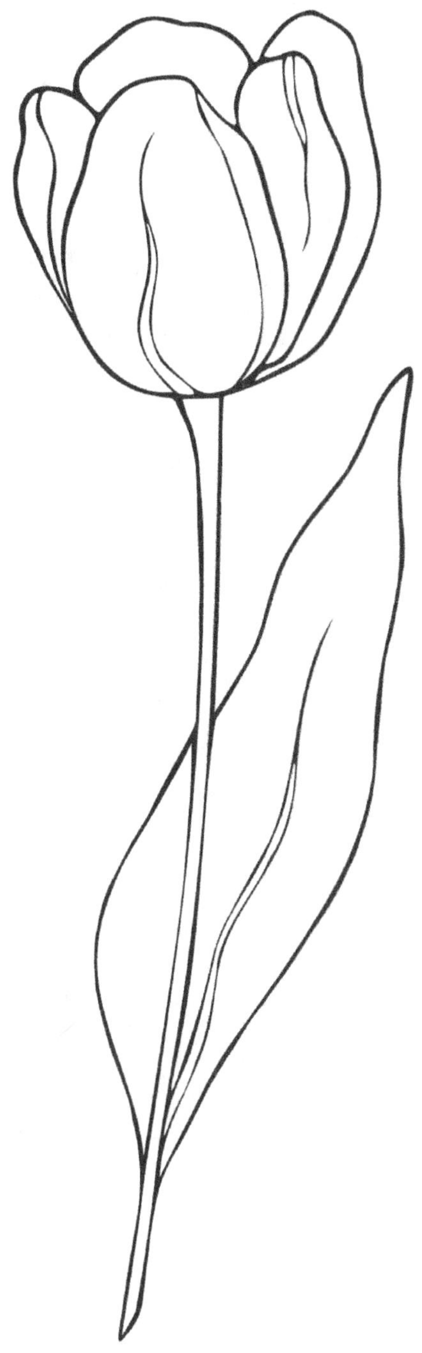

© 2024 - My Peace of Health, LLC

© 2024 - My Peace of Health, LLC

Chapter 1

Embracing Womanhood

I want to talk about something that is truly and utterly awesome. We're all writing the story of our womanhood, and at every moment, with every decision we make, we're choosing our words and what to say next. From the moment we are born, it's like they say, 'Here's your pen, start writing.' As you journey through life, you weave together a tapestry rich with threads of colors, emotions, and experiences of fear, pain, love, and hope. One moment, you may find yourself riding a rollercoaster of emotions, and the next, navigating an unexpected circumstance.

But there's something else all women share that defies their differences. At one level, we may never really know what it means to be a mother, daughter, sister, friend, or laborer. But something, a thread so palpable that it must be real, connects the stories of all of us women. This makes us united in something like a secret sisterhood, bound by more than a shared script.

And isn't it wonderful that the Bible has so much to say about womanhood as well? Proverbs 31:25-26 tells us: 'She is clothed with strength and dignity; she can laugh at the days to come. She speaks with wisdom, and faithful instruction is on her tongue.' Aren't those nice words? Encouraging? A reminder of our strength, our wisdom, our grace?

And then there's Psalm 46:5: 'God is within her, she will not fall; God will help her at break of day.' Girls Power, much? God will help her during the break of the day. Not exactly a throwaway mention, hey.

But you know what makes my heart happy? Kind of like a real-life Wonder Woman story. Have you ever heard of Wilma Rudolph? She's this total powerhouse who overcame some serious odds to become one of the greatest athletes of all time. She got three gold medals at the Olympics. And she did it after a doctor said she would never walk again as a kid. Like, she was, literally, never going to walk again.

© 2024 - My Peace of Health, LLC

But who could be cooler than that? Wilma wasn't just any ole relic in the history books. She was family. More specifically, she was my cousin. Think about it: what could be more empowering than knowing you're related to a three-time winning Olympic champion? That there's a little Wilma, an inherited sense of strength and courage and grace, coursing through your veins?

So, as we dive into this chapter on embracing womanhood with all its highs and lows, victories and defeats, let's remember the incredible legacy of women like Wilma Rudolph. Let's draw inspiration from their stories of resilience, determination, and unwavering faith as we navigate our journeys through womanhood. And hey, who knows? Maybe one day, someone will be telling our stories too.

Navigating roles and responsibilities with confidence.

Balancing the various roles of being a woman, mom, wife, daughter, friend, and professional can often feel like spinning plates. Inevitably, we may occasionally find ourselves dropping a few of them along the way.

However, here is the lovely truth: even when we are bravely balancing many "plates", we possess the power and perseverance to do so with poise and calmness. The trick is finding a way to get everything done with a sense of ease, even as we savor life's joyous offerings with the presence of mind to remain true to ourselves.

That age-old expression 'You can't pour from an empty cup' rings true – and even Jesus retired for a time to recharge and pray in solitude (Mark 1:35). Why wouldn't he? When we empty ourselves, there's nothing left to give. Self-care is not selfish – it keeps our cup full so that we can love and care for others.

Communication, of course, is the other side of this coin. Jesus was, above all else, a master storyteller, dispensing wisdom and truth through all kinds of parables that his audience could readily grasp (eg, Mark 12:37).

And then there's confidence: as long as your faith is in God, and your eyes are on His plan for you, then you can live out life boldly and without

© 2024 - My Peace of Health, LLC

fear because, according to Proverbs 3:26, as long as you're leaning on Him, He'll lead you right and as Philippians 4:13 states, when God is in it, you can do all that you need to do, and you can do all that you want to do.

So, as we wind our way through the hectic mess of life — as we choose the dress to wear, pack the diaper bag, sell the home, prep the children for what's to come, and prepare to settle elsewhere in this transient world — may we do it all with strength and a whole lot of faith that, with God's help, we can weather anything this life puts before us.

Cultivating self-love and inner peace.

I had long dreamed of becoming a woman – the height of beauty, power, and poise. Ever since I can remember, most of my energy as a kid went towards figuring out how to get the high-heeled walk down, then curling my lashes perfectly, and finally learning to blow-dry and curl my hair. When my brother practiced his moonwalk, I mimicked the women around me. If you were an older lady, I most likely studied, copied, and imitated everything you did.

But hanging with the 'big girls' became my full-time job. I was determined to fit in with them. You may remember that old parental question: 'If your friends all jumped off a bridge, would you?' I would reply: 'Yes' (of course, if they were all bungee-jumping!). My premature impulse to grow up fast, combined with my adolescent incompetence, got me into trouble more than a few times.

I thought I was more aware and smarter and I confused that with being mature – which it was not. I was watching 90's music videos and, worse yet, the idea of womanhood that was advanced in sitcoms. None of that represents reality.

Soon enough, that distortion became my reality, and motherhood preceded even my first taste of womanhood, never mind college, or a career, or even an understanding of who I was and what I was meant to be.

© 2024 - My Peace of Health, LLC

I had my son when I was 16 years old. Despite all of my joy being there and all of the excitement of such an incredible event, I was scared out of my mind. Everything I did scared me. Everything I had to do scared me. If only I lived my life the way that I thought God wanted me to live my life, it was shameful – being afraid was shameful, because I had chosen to have my son. It was like I had this scarlet letter 'A' protruding proudly out of my chest for everyone to see, and it was like it stood out proudly for God to see.

Meanwhile, I did not want to let my family down. I wanted to stay the good girl I had always thought they wanted me to be. My journey into motherhood was not the kind of woman's life I had dreamt of for myself. During so much turmoil, and all that shame, here's the one thing that kept me going – and grounded me – in the violence of my despair: my love for my little boy.

I was diaper-changing, burping, feeding, and sleepless, feeling like a fish out of water; I had no idea how to be a woman, let alone a mother. I felt so lost like I'd joined a battlefield without any armor or weapons… Every day I was struggling to simply ease through the chaos. When could I consider myself both a woman and a mother?

Womanhood, once a source of excitement, now felt like a burden. It felt empty, a deep hole that I feared exposing to the world. So, instead of confronting it head-on, I buried it deep within myself, hoping that by hiding it away, I could somehow mask my insecurities and shortcomings.

But as the years went on and I lived through the rollercoaster of mom life, something happened. A strength, a resilience, a still, small voice, started to emerge from somewhere deep within me, an inner light that could never be stifled.

The hardship of being a mother was a revelation for me. I learned that the most feminine thing is often not the loud, imperious declaration of one's needs; perhaps it is the quiet persistence and sticking with things. I saw that, for me at least, dignity had more to do with respecting my actual self – with all of its imperfections – with courage and downright bravery and not with pretending to be how I thought I should be nor what I was not.

© 2024 - My Peace of Health, LLC

And grace — that's what I was craving so badly when I was racked with pent-up shame and guilt for my actions. Then, as soon as I surrendered my self-inflicted wounds to something greater than me, that's when I finally understood what grace was. God forgave me. I was flooded with unconditional love. And I was given the grace to walk in truth.

I look at my scars today, as I embrace mid-life, and I stand in wonder and thanksgiving. I no longer cringe. I no longer feel ashamed. I look upon my scars, the living scars of pain, and I remember that they are treasures of grace and that those who are redeemed are not those who are without flaws – we are those who are perfectly flawed. I walk today, not with a heavy conscience that comes with embarrassment, but with a heart that knows I am fearfully and wonderfully made as a redeemed child of God.

With that in mind, let's begin addressing this all-important practice of loving, accepting, and finding peace with ourselves.

That voice that says: 'You are not enough,' we always need to find a counter voice to it, a deep well of self-acceptance-how many people can love and care for others when they are not honoring their own life?

I want to tell you a story about a woman I've come to think of as a good friend, Yolanda. Yolanda is the mother of six children, and that, by itself, would have afforded her a lifetime of emotional labor. But Yolanda is also a survivor, a victim of domestic violence at a point where, understandably, she wondered if the struggle would kill her.

When God rescued her from that, he delivered her from her husband, sure, but he then began delivering her from the wounds inflicted upon her – 'by his stripes were we healed.' Isaiah 53:5 The road to healing was a long one, and the months and years were full of ups and downs, times of faith, and times of doubt and fear. But each step, it seemed, was marked by peace, that not one of us could comprehend– at least not fully – a peace that passeth understanding, only needing to flow from the arms of her Heavenly Father.

I have had the privilege of witnessing Yolanda's growth, day by day, and how she has taken hold of her life and experiences. I have seen her rise

© 2024 - My Peace of Health, LLC

from the ashes of her former life. I have witnessed the peace within her. And believe me when I say that she has never been more alive. Amen.

Her story reminds us that no matter how badly we've been hurt, no matter how broken we might be or how dirty we might feel, there is deep and enduring healing for our wounds. It stresses that the greatest work in our lives is our own and happens through the practice of loving ourselves, accepting ourselves, and finding peace within us. It stems from inviting God's light into our darkness and allowing Him to bring us, in our entirety, into a place of healing.

Knowing that you'll learn from Yolanda's story, stand a little taller in your skin, and open your heart a little wider to the gifts of your personality. It takes courage to be vulnerable, to embrace something beautiful, that stirs deeply within. But most of all, I hope that you embrace a deep well of self-acceptance, self-love, and, of course, self-forgiveness. You are fearfully and wonderfully made. You were beautifully and marvelously put together. You were created in the image of a loving God.

Having walked this path with many women in a myriad of ways, I want to guide you through this legacy of learning while pointing to an even richer heritage, the wisdom of Scripture.

We previously discussed the significance of self-love – of loving ourselves enough to find clarity and peace about the power given to us by God. We will examine the same questions from our biblical examples in this section. We'll see how women in Scripture embodied strength, dignity, and purpose.

Having opened up the biblical treasures of stories and teachings about women, we now turn our gaze back to the present moment. Where are we now as women of faith? What have we discovered that can encourage us in our ongoing faith adventures?

1. Strength and Resilience:

© 2024 - My Peace of Health, LLC

From Proverbs 31:25-26: Strength and dignity are her clothing, And she smiles at the future. She opens her mouth in wisdom, And on her tongue is instruction. And because Strength and dignity are hers; She smiles at the future. She opens her mouth in wisdom, And the teaching of kindness is on her tongue strength and dignity are yours. You are beautiful, confident, strong, and dignified. You can laugh at the future because you are grounded in wisdom and faithful instruction is on your tongue.

She was an orphan of Jewish ancestry – a person in exile – yet Esther gave a display of exemplary bravery in putting her life on the line to prevent the annihilation of her people, trusting that obedience to God's plan would enable her to endure the most terrible of circumstances, even when it would cost her everything. Her story affirms for all time and circumstances that God can indeed work with common women to fulfill his extraordinary purposes in the execution of his good plan.

2. Compassion and Empathy:

Then there's the unforgettable account, from Luke 10:38-42, of the sisters Martha and Mary who received our Lord Jesus in their home. They have different ways of expressing calm and compassion to stay connected. Unlike Martha who's busily running around preparing (we can well identify with that, too!), Mary is sitting at Jesus' feet listening to him speak. The Lord commends Mary, choosing the 'better' part, over Martha's 'anxiety' (another word that captures some of the challenges of our time) induced busyness.

An example of the increasing care that Jesus extended to women is told in John 4:1-42. In the story of the woman at the well, Jesus ignores the first and most obvious boundary: that between male and female. And, having come to a well in a town that is desolate or forgotten by the authorities and assigned as a suitable place for women who have been sent away or judged as outsiders – Samaritans in John 4 – he will then be positioned to offer the Samaritan woman, her community and her listeners the possibility of a new way of living, fulfilled in the Messiah. A compassion that grasps what was required to overcome barriers with the poor, marginalized, and outcast women becomes inclusive compassion for all people on the margins of polite society and orthodox religious life.

© 2024 - My Peace of Health, LLC

3. Wisdom and Leadership:

Besides Psalms, the wisdom literature of the Bible (Proverbs, for example, and Ecclesiastes) contains some wonderful insights for women who want to learn how to live out their faith in their daily lives. Proverbs 31:30 reads: 'Charm is deceitful, and beauty is vain, but a woman who fears the Lord is to be praised.'

Judges 4-5 tells the story of Deborah, judge and prophetess, who defies a male-dominated society to lead Israel into a battle against its enemies. Deborah shows her courageous leadership, proving that God can use women in leadership roles and to affect change.

4. Grace and Redemption:

A beautiful example of this grace is found in John 8:1-11, the well-known story of the woman caught in adultery: As Jesus straightened up and saw her, he said, 'Woman, where are they? Has no one condemned you?' She said, 'No one, sir.' And Jesus said, 'Neither do I condemn you. Go now and leave your life of sin.' Jesus could have condemned her to death, yet he did not. She was guilty, yet he forgave her and welcomed her into a new way of living. This is God's grace and redemption – that there is no one God cannot forgive.

The Apostle Paul's teachings on one's unity in Christ, like Galatians 3:28, emphasizes that all human beings – women included – are equally valued before God: 'There is neither Jew nor Gentile, neither slave nor free, nor is there male and female, for you are all one in Christ Jesus.' Here, Paul asserts the equality of all who believe in Christ: slaves, women, Jews, and Gentiles.

So, what does it look like when these biblical principles are applied to the challenges and experiences that are common to women today, both then and now? How do you embody your calling as a daughter of God? What do you have to offer the world?

The pitfalls for women in society, as I've already alluded to, are many and varied. Our confidence in the identity and purpose that Christ offers can be shaken by the cravings of our flesh – the voice that tells us we're

© 2024 - My Peace of Health, LLC

not thin enough, pretty enough or smart enough. By now, you probably know that this voice isn't just the result of any one environment or challenge. Its origins are as Biblical as the nature of God himself. Your fearful and wondrous God, like the generous and loving father who He always intended to be, has always wanted to be known, yet known intimately. And so, generations on from the women we've read about, women today can take heart. We too can embrace our calling today as the daughters of God. We too, can know what it feels like to hold the power and purpose that He offers.

But these pressures and struggles – and the way we navigate them – are all reminders that womanhood goes much deeper than the outside perceptions and expectations that the world can foist upon us. Recognizing that we exist as daughters of God, valued and deeply loved, is a source of strength we can use to face up to and overcome the challenges we may experience. And yet, there is a baseline reality: if we struggle as daughters of God, much of that will necessarily intersect with our physical and spiritual health. From the teen years to the transition through menopause – and beyond – our wellbeing, as both a physical and spiritual responsibility, should be approached with purpose, intention, and self-care.

Reproductive Health

Let's view reproductive health as our body's best friend, a constant companion that guides us through the ups and downs of life. Think of a journey. Each phase brings its own set of experiences, challenges, and joy. The teen years are a time to get to know our bodies better; learn about menstruation, and maybe tackle PCOS or other conditions. As we grow older, we continue this journey, with more emphasis on birth control, family planning, pregnancy, and the excitement (or dread!) that brings. However, we need to be alert to the fact that STIs and fibroids may pop up, unannounced. And menopause, a phase of hormonal shifts and transitions, is waiting for us, like a roller coaster ride that we might as well take together. Knowledge, a supportive community, and self-care can help us navigate this journey, with confidence and girl power.

© 2024 - My Peace of Health, LLC

Reproductive health is part of our womanhood journey, after all, and it reflects the many stages of identity and role formation that we cover in this chapter. As with womanhood, some aspects of reproductive health will be effortless, and some will feel more arduous. There will be disappointments and celebrations, uncertainties and triumphs. But we can face them bravely and boldly with the spirit and courage that this chapter encourages, because to be a woman is to be strong, no matter if you are at the beginning of life, in your prime, or at the other end of the spectrum. Let's continue our conversation about reproductive health with openness, support, and a reaffirmation of the ever-present interconnectedness between our womanhood journey and reproductive health.

Pregnancy and Childbirth

There's nothing like mom life. Don't get it twisted. If mom's life isn't for you, have no fear. Your role is simply to bask in the live footage, to sit back and take in the birth. And then take a breath of relief that it's not you. 'Cause what a ride, eh? From the first flutters to the first cries, it's an adventure the whole way through! So we celebrate every step. From that first kick to that placenta, you're creating new life, aren't you?

True, pregnancy can be a tad bit, agonizing. There's the morning sickness, the backache, the nausea. But isn't all that a small price to pay for bringing so much joy into the world? And surely, when we release our babies into this world, we'll be surrounded by loved ones, our family, and friends who will help us while they wake up with tears of happiness. It will be completely different from any experience we've ever had before when, indeed, something new is born. The miraculous nature of pregnancy and birth can be placed in the same reverential scientific category as all the moments that led to the Universe's creation. Pregnancy and birth are the recreation of the Universe.

© 2024 - My Peace of Health, LLC

Navigating Menopause

Sailing through menopause: it's like another ride, we still don't have a seat belt to hold on to …The most common complaint attributed to menopause is hot flashes. More than half of the women in the study experienced hot flushes, which appear to increase as estrogen levels drop. Some women describe hot flashes as a 'wash of heat' or 'dripping sweat', usually important during the night and is one of the most debilitating symptoms of menopause.

No one is one hundred percent immune to the side effects of menopause: hot flashes and night sweats, mood swings, and sleep disturbances. And yet, a marker of a woman's body moving from one stage of life through to the next, menopause is a rite of passage as well as a road map, one worth traveling.

But, let's face menopause straight on, with the candid maturity, entertainment, and dry humor we've surely earned with all the storms that have come and gone before this one. With the support of each other, with proper self-care, and maybe some good laughs along the way, we'll master menopause and come out the other side the same glorious boss babes we were going in.

Prioritizing Preventive Screenings:

Focusing on preventive screenings is our way of giving ourselves the gift of health – of stepping ahead of the game. It's like keeping the body well-lubricated, like a well-tuned machine.

Screening for example, for breast and cervical cancer via mammograms and Pap smears, helps us stay ahead of the disease and prevent cancer from ever developing. It gives us reassurance that we are proactively taking care of ourselves and catching any problems before they develop.

Ok, so it's not exactly fun to set all those appointments up – but it's a huge payoff for you and your future. Invest in yourself if you want to carry on living your life "happy and healthy or something".

© 2024 - My Peace of Health, LLC

Therefore make a vow to attend our preventive screenings! Let's show up for ourselves and each other. Our lives are precious! And together, we can do this!

As we close this chapter on womanhood, I hope we carry with us the wisdom, strength, and grace we read about together. Sisters, let us hold onto this understanding: our story is made up of many experiences, some difficult and discouraging, some joyful and triumphant, but threaded through with grace, compassion, and deep faith. Let us hold onto each other as we make our way forward, climbing mountains and descending valleys, knowing that we are indeed 'fearfully and wonderfully made' and cared for by 'the eyes of God' (Psalm 21:15). Are you strong enough to live out your calling as a daughter of God? If not, what steps can you take to develop that self-love and inner peace that you so desperately need? And as you make those changes, know that you are not alone. Dozens of women before you have walked through the trial you are facing. Study their lives. Learn from their advice and examples. Let your story of womanhood be written, not with guilt, shame, pain, or defeat, but with hope, courage, grace, and resolution that God has a purpose for your life.

We must live out our stories as women in the world, battered, bruised, in pain, and with scars, and it will be a legacy that is beautiful, powerful, and the most wonderful gift we can give to our daughters, our granddaughters, and the generations of women who will come after us. My greatest hope is that this chapter has left you feeling more motivated and stronger than you have ever been before. I will leave you all with one final piece of wisdom: 'Be strong and courageous. Do not be afraid or terrified because of them, for the Lord your God goes with you; he will never leave you nor forsake you.' ~ Deuteronomy 31:6

© 2024 - My Peace of Health, LLC

Discussion Questions:

1. What does womanhood mean to you? How has your understanding changed throughout your life?

2. Have you ever experienced guilt or shame about being a woman? How did you manage that?

© 2024 - My Peace of Health, LLC

3. What sorts of strength and resilience do you see in the women around you, whether they're in your immediate circle or at large?

4. How do you make space for rest and renewal amid your busy life? What are your practices for finding peace, grounding, and resilience within yourself?

5. Think of a woman from history, literature, or your own life whom you respect for her courage, dignity, and grace. What traits do you most admire about her – and how do they speak to your own experiences?

© 2024 - My Peace of Health, LLC

© 2024 - My Peace of Health, LLC

© 2024 - My Peace of Health, LLC

© 2024 - My Peace of Health, LLC

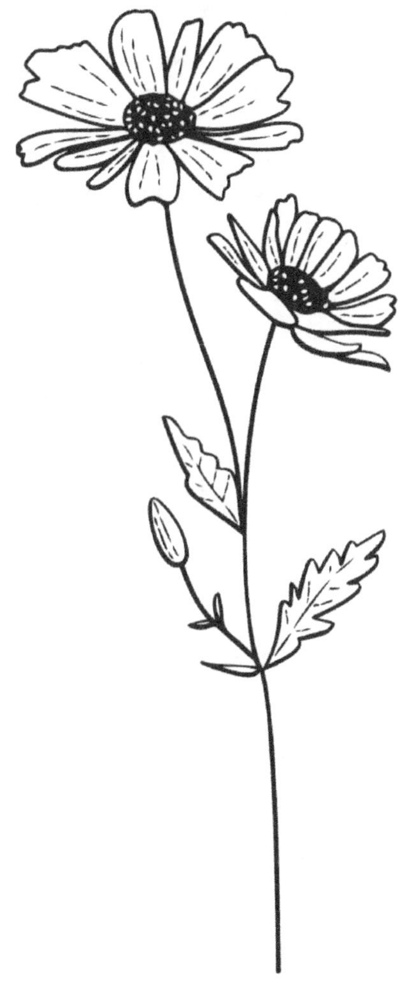

© 2024 - My Peace of Health, LLC

Chapter 2

Nourishing Body and Mind

We are so engrossed in the day-to-day tasks and multitude of details of ourselves. We have to stop. Need to stop – really. This is so much bigger than us. All this self-care stuff we do – it is not just for us; our families need to grow and flourish with us – and there just isn't much go-slow in this go, go, go world. You have to try and make space for your bodies and brains and souls. Real wellness? It isn't about the quick fix and isn't about the trend of the moment. It is about balance and about being our radiant selves.

Our bodies are the greatest gifts that God could give us. They are supposed to be cherished gifts and they should be cherished. Did not Paul say that the body is the temple of the Holy Spirit? 1 Cor 6:19-20. We are supposed to be nice to our bodies.

But wellness is a much bigger deal than any of the talk about the physical stuff. It's about going to the deep places of the mind and soul, learning about the insides of us as much as the outsides. Do you remember that verse from Romans 12:2? 'Do not be conformed to this world, but be transformed by the renewal of your minds'? Yeah, that kind of thing.

And let me tell you, I've witnessed the beauty of holistic wellness firsthand. It's not so much checking boxes as it is intentionally creating life – a life purposefully created to feed every cell in our body and every fiber of our soul.

Practical Tips for Holistic Wellness:

With that in mind, here are some simple, gentle ways to start:

- Start small: Don't abandon small things and insist on massive changes, but embrace baby steps instead, and celebrate every mini-win.

© 2024 - My Peace of Health, LLC

- Go for it: But keep your goals realistic, and within your reach. Make goals that you can achieve.
- Don't beat yourself up: We're human after all, things happen, and it is what it is. Learn from it.
- Surround yourself with your people: those who love you and who you can love in return – friends, family, a community of like-minded individuals. You need to be supported.
- Stay close to your why: always remember the reason you are on the wellness path anyway – for you, for the family, or beyond.

These practical tips are steps that you can take to realize the more general framework for wellness that I've discussed above.

Healthy Eating:

Now, for one of the most common obstacles: healthy eating. Stress, busy schedules, and an abundance of junk food make it difficult to maintain nutritious eating habits, but here's the real secret: getting the whole family involved. The family can become fully engaged in menu planning and food preparation, and you will shift your entire mindset about eating. When cooking becomes a family activity, not only do we take greater control over how, when, and what we eat, but we also help our children build healthy habits.

Benefits of a Plant-Based Diet:

So, the first thing is to look at the pros of becoming herbivorous. We know from research that using a large amount of fruits, vegetables, whole grains, beans, nuts and seeds in the diet will generate major health improvements, as is recommended in such books as How Not to Die by Dr Michael Greger, can make you feel amazing, and can be great for your health.

Now, let's break down the incredible benefits of focusing on plant-based foods:

- **Nutrient-Rich Foods:** The health-giving, anti-disease foods. Yes, I'm talking about the vitamin, mineral, and fiber-rich foods,

© 2024 - My Peace of Health, LLC

the energy and health-givers. Think rainbows and green pastures.

- **Heart Health:** The facts couldn't be any clearer: plant foods are great for your heart. You won't need to keep a defibrillator and nitroglycerin pills handy. No more dread wondering whether the doctor is going to take your cholesterol or blood pressure. When you put the plants front and center and take the animals a few steps back, your heart gets some plant love, and you lower the chance that it is going to give you any hiccups.
- **Digestive Health:** Fiber is like a big bear hug for your tummy, helping to keep everything moving and helping you to say 'buh-bye' to bloating and constipation. Get some fibrous fruits, vegetables, whole grains, and legumes into your life, and your tummy will be giving you a big thanks.
- **Weight Management:** Plant-based diets are like your BFF when it comes to weight management! Low in calories and saturated fats but high in fiber? Yes, please! When you're filling up on nutrient-rich plant foods, you're naturally keeping your calories in check longer, and maximizing your satiation – this is heaven for your waistline!
- **Environmental Sustainability**: You're not only blessing your health but also honoring God's creation! Plant-based diets carry a divine touch, with a significantly smaller environmental impact compared to those laden with animal products. So, by extending a warm welcome to more plants and gently bidding farewell to those animal delights, you're not only nurturing your body but also embracing your stewardship role on this Earth, giving thanks to the Creator for His abundant gifts.

Toast to plants, the truest fast food! By following a plant-based diet, you are not only feeding your body, but you are feeding your soul, and you are ensuring a more sustainable, happier, and healthier world for all.

Armed with this information, you're now empowered to use plant-based foods to steer your growing family in the right direction. Here's how to get started.

© 2024 - My Peace of Health, LLC

1. **Colorful Variety**: Time to spice up dinner with colorful fruit and veggies! It's not just about eating right, it's about setting the table for an adventure! Grab your entire crew and take the plunge into learning new flavors and textures.
2. **Whole Grains**: Hello, whole grains – brown rice, quinoa and oats! Put down your breadsticks and make room for these energy-packed grains, which also contain fiber to fill you up. It's easy to cook these up, so why not make a noodle quinoa dish or swap the pasta in your favorite family recipes with whole grains?
3. **Plant Proteins:** Get bodybuilding with family-feeding plant proteins! Nuts and seeds, legumes and beans – and tofu, too! – all have flavor and … uh, nutrition for your gang. Make meal prep a family entertainment event as you prepare a delicious and nutritious protein creation for your gang.
4. **Cut Out Processed Foods:** Whole foods, minimally processed, were designed to work with our body, not against it. As a family, read the labels together and purchase what will feed your body well on the inside.
5. **Stay Hydrated:** Stay hydrated for a great night's sleep. Energy and nourishment from water, inside and out, help you keep your glow. Keep away from sugary drinks and get infused waters and homemade smoothies instead.

Here are fun tips guaranteed to turn plant-power eating from a great experiment to a delicious map to flavourful fun and fabulous family health.

Exercise for Overall Health:

And what about exercise? You've probably heard it all before… cardio, strength training, and stretching – whatever form of exercise you choose, it is extremely important to keep your heart and body healthy. If you're not sure how to get started, ask your doctor for an exercise prescription to guide you, or hire a trainer to keep you accountable.

Not that you should work out merely for good health. But consider each rep a praise song to God because of the body He's blessed you with and the ability to walk, run, lift, or participate in a fitness class.

© 2024 - My Peace of Health, LLC

And then there are the virtues of fitness: grit, patience, and resilience. All the qualities of our faith – as the Bible teaches – and demands that we possess. Getting through that interval workout? That's not just about building biceps, it's about building the soul, too.

A reminder, your body is a temple, and a gift from God. As you tie your shoes or pick up your dumbbells for your workout, you're not working out — you're worshiping with each sweat session. We are to be good stewards of our bodies, using them for whatHe created them for, and honoring Him in all that we do with them.

Here are some easy family fitness tips:

Get Your Move On: Go for walks, bike rides, play backyard soccer, or have a living-room dance party. Find activities that all can share and enjoy. Do these often.

 Set Family Fitness Goals: Come up with goals together (eg, reaching 10,000 steps each day, or learning a new sport together). Keep track of your progress as a family, and celebrate when the whole family achieves their goals.

Try Outdoor Fun: Take a hike. Swim. Have a picnic. Play on the beach. Outdoor recreation provides endless opportunities for family fitness fun.

Make Playtime Active: Set up a game of tag, hopscotch, or Simon Says and get kids moving. Make play time active and add a dash of creativity to keep kids on their feet.

Show them the way: You are your children's role model. So get fit yourself. Whether it's exercising by jogging in the morning, going to the gym, or even riding your bike, bring them with you and let them share in your activities.

Transitioning to stress management, let's explore how we can tackle stress together.

Stress Management:

© 2024 - My Peace of Health, LLC

Alright, let's tackle stress head-on! First, create a healthy daily rhythm that includes stress-relieving activities — deep breathing exercises, family naps, and anything that can bring a bit of relaxation to your day and make it more enjoyable.

1. Make your home sanctuary a place for peaceful downtime by spending some time each day doing something restorative and relaxing as a family, such as reading, drawing, or listening to gentle music.
2. Communicate! Communicate! Communicate! Create an atmosphere where everyone feels safe to share, ask questions, offer feedback, and talk about their feelings. Be an active listener and listen with empathy to provide each other with mutual support in difficult moments.

So here I am, coming into the Wells home with the family of four – they're on the go. Busy, busy – but they wanted more of the good stuff, you know? They wanted more calm and connection, and to truly feel connected in their homes, which is great – that's what I am here to provide.

We started this journey together, exploring practices to nurture their mental and spiritual well-being. We took inspiration from scripture but made it easy to serve this modern family, creating a recipe for family harmony that would make even Martha Stewart jealous.

Denise would send me texts every morning about how they finally had gathered for prayer and devotion, and they felt more prepared in their spirits for whatever the Lord had in store for them that day. She'd tell me about their workout sessions for the week, how they lifted one another – in the truest sense of the word.

By evening, they would be reading each other portions of their love journals, cultivating a kind of intimacy right in the living room; and, over the weekend, I'd receive photographs of them outdoors, smiles wide, nestled in a blanket.

© 2024 - My Peace of Health, LLC

Watching the Wells transform was a sight to behold. Tensions eased, conversations flowed, and their home became a sanctuary of love and acceptance.

Once the Wells had begun to move towards overall wellness, the changes in their family were dramatic. Gone was the tension that had been eating away at their home day in and day out. Instead, their home often overflowed with laughter. As their marriage improved, so did the rest of their house. "The atmosphere is much different," Denise told me. "We can talk more." So can the children. And then there is sleep.

And now – their minds and hearts settled and restored – the Wells family embrace healthy sleep as a pillar of integrated wellness, prioritizing a balanced sleep routine and a comfortable bedtime environment, knowing that a restorative night's sleep is critical for physical, mental, and emotional restoration.

In the evening, they read aloud together as a family, prayed together, or ate together while expressing gratitude for the evening's blessings. The lights were dimmed or turned off, and the TV was shut off to minimize distractions from the natural winding-down process that prepares the body for sleep. Whenever possible, work stress was left at the door.

As each night passed, the Wells found themselves reaping the benefits of sleep hygiene, getting up refreshed and ready to meet the day, for they had begun the process of rewriting corrective sleep into their lives – lines that flowed through both mind and body.

Amidst the sounds of their sleep sanctuary, the Wells family not only recharged their physical batteries and deepened their sense of connection and rhythm but also were one step closer to achieving their long-term healing goals through sleep. True healing happens inside and out. It is this metabolization that ignites the spirit and brings new light and life to every corner of our reality.

Importance of Quality Sleep in Holistic Wellness

Everything's better when you get a good night's sleep. At night, while you're between the sheets, your cells are rejuvenating, your brain is

© 2024 - My Peace of Health, LLC

consolidating the day's experiences, and your mood gets to have a timeout. When you don't get good sleep, your general well-being suffers.

Good sleep is important for your health and well-being. Here is how you can improve your sleep:

1. Keep a Regular Sleep Schedule: Go to bed and get up at the same time every day of the week (this includes weekends).
2. Have a Wind-Down Ritual: Set a relaxing bedtime ritual, such as having a book before bed or taking a warm bath, that clues your brain and body into time for winding down.
3. Turn Off Screens: Avoid using smartphones, tablets, or computers for at least an hour before bed because the blue light that they emit keeps you alert.
4. Your Caffeine and Alcohol Intake: Avoid caffeine and alcohol during the evening time frame since they inhibit sleep initiation and will disrupt your sleep patterns.

Try these and you'll enjoy better sleep and better health.

Addressing Common Sleep Disturbances:

1. **Insomnia**: If you have insomnia or otherwise have trouble sleeping, relaxation techniques are a good idea. And of course, you want to avoid arousing activities or substances right before bedtime, as you do in any successful state of sleep. If you have insomnia then make sure to discuss it with your health services provider.
1. **Sleep Apnea**: If you are worried you have obstructive sleep apnea with loud snoring or excessive daytime sleepiness, see your healthcare provider and consider evaluation and treatment with continuous positive airway pressure (CPAP) therapy or lifestyle modifications.
1. **Restless Legs Syndrome (RLS):** While sometimes simple lifestyle changes such as altering your bedtime routine or adding relaxation techniques make a significant difference, the key thing is to not let restless legs interfere with your sleep. If you have restless legs, share your concerns with your doctor.

© 2024 - My Peace of Health, LLC

2. **Nightmares:** Relaxation techniques before bedtime, with deep breathing or meditation on scriptures, can help quiet your mind enough to let sleep overtake you. Sensory experiences inside your bedroom that are pleasant and comforting, like soft lighting, have also been shown to reduce the occurrence of nightmares.

To sum up, let sleep hygiene become an important part of your holistic wellness journey. Make sure to have a healthy sleep routine, master the right bedtime environment, and deal with the common sleep issues in the right way, to maximize your sleep quality and support your pursuit towards holistic wellness. Sleep health is self-care, and good sleep health is a healthful investment you commit to yourself to secure your happiness.

In other words, this chapter on nurturing the body and mind is not the final one on the journey to holistic wellness, which is a long-distance race. Focus on the small daily victories, the baby steps taken toward better balance, and the attention given to feeding the flesh, mind, and spirit.

If you focus on enjoying nutritious foods and are physically active, manage your stress and engage in mindfulness practices, and take steps to improve your sleep through good sleep hygiene, then you're helping to ensure not just a healthy body now, but a happy, healthy you in the future.

So cheers to self-care, to your wonderful path of healing and wellness ahead, and, most importantly, cheers to you. You are already doing it, and I'm toasting you all the way home.

And now on to the exercises! I hope to make these explorations of the self as playful and enjoyable as possible. After all, we only have one!

© 2024 - My Peace of Health, LLC

Interactive Exercises:

Let's make this journey of self-discovery and wellness enhancement fun and engaging! Here are some interactive exercises and reflection prompts to dive into:

1. **Wellness Check-In**: Are you checking in on yourself? Rate your current wellness practices: from 1 (worst) to 10 (best). Where are you strongest in your physical, mental, and spiritual wellness? What areas need improvement?

2. **Goal Setting Galore:** Choose a wellness goal for each of your three indicators of wellness (physical body, mental health, spiritual well-being), and then write down each. Make your goals specific and measurable, and come up with a series of action steps that you can take towards it. Then, try to spend a reasonable amount of time on each.

© 2024 - My Peace of Health, LLC

3. **Daily Gratitude Journal:** Get a journal or notebook and add five things each day that you are thankful for. Perhaps one of the first principles, if not the first, of many religions and cultures in the world is the idea of gratitude, and this practice can be so amazing for your well-being in life because it can help you shift your perception of life (and can also be all sorts of surprising and inspiring, too!)

4. **Scripture Reflection:** Pick out a scripture verse or quote from a notable spiritual leader or stream of thought that most ignites your spirit. Read it, then reflect on it. How does this resonate with you? How can you apply these words to how you move through your day? Journal your reflections or discuss them with a trusted friend or mentor to explore more about how this makes sense in your life.

© 2024 - My Peace of Health, LLC

© 2024 - My Peace of Health, LLC

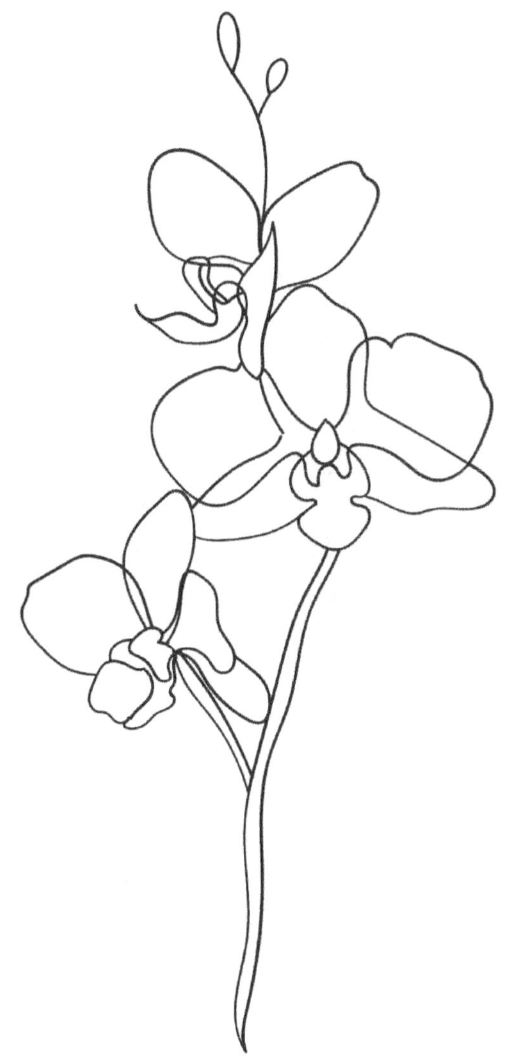

© 2024 - My Peace of Health, LLC

© 2024 - My Peace of Health, LLC

Chapter 3

Building Strong Relationships

Wait, wait. Don't put down this book quite yet. You need to know this: the single biggest predictor of wellness is relationship – and this chapter alone will have your name written all over it whether you are single, partnered, or parented. Solo or pair, this stuff is highly relevant and there is gold to be found here. Read on and become a happier, healthier you through your most powerful relationships.

Marriage and Partnership:

Let's get married (or partnered)! Let's get on this exciting ride! It'll go up and down (and upside-down), and you'll hold on tight to each other through the turns; you'll lean on each other for support, and that's what bonding is all about.

Back in the day, I had two little ones tagging along, and I was embracing life's whirlwind ride. Whatever man God had for me – him I was destined to meet, not just a lover, but a mate, a partner, and a man who feared God.

Enter Simon, my knight in shining armor (or in this case, in a hoodie and jeans). When we crossed paths at my ripe old age of 21, I knew I had found him: someone who was not just another check on my wish list but an ardent lover of God who had a heart as vast as the sky, and a genuine desire to build a God-centered home.

I will never pretend our relationship has been easy. I can tell you that it hasn't. We've had bumpy rides, choppy seas, and wave after wave has threatened to break us up. Talking has sometimes proved problematic. What can I say?

During all of this, there has been one constant: our mission towards God. I am constantly reminded that love is a choice; loving is a daily decision to die to myself and choose to love, even when I don't 'feel' the warm fuzzies.

© 2024 - My Peace of Health, LLC

And having a loving God available to us has, in deed and truth, made all the difference when it comes to fighting and hurting feelings and disappointed expectations.

Now, here's the good part: becoming a happy couple reduces your risk of disease and even death: married couples, especially those who are happily married, are less stressed, and have better heart health and even immune systems, compared with those who are single. It creates a real near-magical health and mood boost.

But let's not sugarcoat it either. Real marriage is not always easy. There are as many days of wrestling as there are cuddling. And you know what? It's OK. Because of those challenges? They are growth opportunities, for closeness, for the love that lasts.

Having a loving God along for the ride has made all the difference – especially in life's disagreements, hurts, and disappointments.

So here's the bottom line, on your journey through marriage's beautiful mess, remember this:

1. **Prioritize Connection:** be determined to spend more time with them, to find out what makes them tick, to share a hobby or make love or talk or listen, or to just be together in the same room and know they are there.
2. **Practice Gratitude:** Gratitude expressed to a partner can create a more positive outlook towards your partner and greater gratitude for your marriage. This effect occurs likely because gratitude directs attention towards the positive aspects of your life, and makes you feel good!
3. **Navigate Conflict with Care**: You're going to have conflicts. The question is, how do you manage them? Figure out how to Agree and Disagree well, through empathy, listening, and thinking about each other as teammates
4. **Invest in Self-Care:** Find the activities that make you happy and do them. Never undermine the power and importance of sleep and rest. There is no shame in getting help if and when you need it.

© 2024 - My Peace of Health, LLC

5. **Go to a couples therapist or counselor if you need to:** For the
    right reason: There are moments when the troubles of a marriage
    could be smoothed out through the intervention of a couples
    therapist or counselor. Don't be ashamed to get help.

It is your greatest wellness benefit in life, immersing yourself into this
life-altering and life-changing adventure of love and marriage, your
marriage will be more than a source of coitus, consolation, and joy; it will
be your greatest wellness benefit. To your health, indeed.

Parent-Child Relationships:

Hang on to your hats, folks, because we're about to drive straight into
the thrill ride of parenting. It's as wonderful and rocky and full of
twisty-turny moments as anything I have ever experienced – and I have
been a mother for what feels like forever. All that messiness adds up to
create this wonderful thing called a child – and in turn, adds up to
complete us and them.

Another news flash: yes, the parent-child tie can affect everyone's health
and happiness for the better. Strong parent-child connections can
decrease stress, increase resilience, and sweeten the entire show.

And so, just for a moment, let us pause over what the Bible says about
family love. We are God's children, and since our Father in heaven loves
us, we are to love and care for our children in that same way.

Home should be a little heaven on earth, full of love, reason, and
kindness. Ephesians 6:4 tells parents to 'bring [your children] up in the
training and instruction of the Lord'. Or in plain English: teach them
what's right and spend every day loving them up.

But hang on – what if you've just had one of those days when you feel
like you dropped the ball in being a parent? I've been there and, frankly,
I've done that: I've got the T-shirt to prove it. Parenting is no picnic – it's
unpredictable, and we're all winging it.

I interrupt this entry with a minor story of shame. My son was getting
ready for a church play and we were pulling out of the driveway when his

© 2024 - My Peace of Health, LLC

sibling yelled that he forgot his shoes in the house. So we went back and, in total meltdown, I ran inside the house, slamming doors and storming around furious, looking for this boy's shoe. Come to find out, his shoes were in the car. FACEPALM. But besides being wrong, I forgot to show him patience and love at that moment. I wasn't treating him like the child of God he is, instead I treated this sweet soul like the enemy. Total shame. This brings me to the minor point that we all fail, but even in times of total failure, God's grace and love are there reminding us what love even looks like.

But here's the thing: those hard parts? That's the job. And even when we mess up, God's grace and love are right there to pick us up and brush us off. And so, when you get that parenting-fails feeling, take a deep breath, friend. All things, including self-forgiveness and restoration? Yep, they're on the table. Just start with giving yourself a little grace, maybe even asking your little one to forgive you when you need to. You got this.

Here's a little plan to help you move forward:

1. **Take a Breather:** Sweet mama, take a breath. Stop. Pause. Give yourself a high five for the wins, a hug for the hard stuff, and throw a party for surviving.
2. **Reach Out:** Sister, I know that it can be tough to do this on your own, so don't feel like you have to. If you need support, go to your village (your girlfriends, your mom's group, spouse, or a counselor) to talk about it.
3. **Forgive Yourself**: Repeat after me: 'I'm human, and I am allowed to mess up.' You deserve to not beat yourself up, girl. Let it go, give yourself a break. You messed up, you let yourself and/or others down. Life goes on, it's a new day – that's a new slate.
4. **Connect with Your Kiddos:** Get down on the floor to color or play legos then settle in for two stories and a hug. This is the good stuff. Let's find some love and laughs along the way!
5. **Keep Growing:** Honey, parenting is a lifelong journey of personal growth. Be open to new ideas and strategies. Learn and grow. And on those days when it feels like nothing is going according to

© 2024 - My Peace of Health, LLC

plan, know that you are doing an amazing job – truly, are you killing it!

Go ahead and celebrate the good days while admitting the bad ones and showering yourself with grace. Pour that love into those little people like there's no tomorrow. Home is a space of love, and that is the most beautiful thing.

Friendship and Community:

There are some interesting things to discuss about adult friendships, aren't there? I'm glad you asked! You have just arrived at an education/coaching class on making friends and building community as an adult. At this point, many who have tried it assume that finding supportive friends is as likely as finding a needle in a haystack. And yet the successful ones have already discovered that it is possible and worthwhile.

Think about the fact that you're an adult now, with adult things to do and adult obligations to fulfill, and, yes, someone who probably isn't scooting along on a bike to a neighbor's house to chat the way that kid's once did. The truth is, while making friends as an adult might take a bit more effort than it used to when we were children, there's no reason that it has to be any less rewarding.

Hey, here's Jesus and His disciples, why don't we follow their example? Jesus didn't call them followers, He called them friends. He expected them to follow Him side-by-side, supporting each other along the way, sticking with Him no matter what, and drawing close to Jesus together.

Life is a wild ride and, on the way, you need a good crew, the ride-or-die friends who pick you up, root for you, and tell you to look up from your feet and look to Jesus.

So, where can you meet friends as an adult? By getting out and about, and saying yes to opportunities to connect with new people. Join a local church or group; attend community activities or festivals; stop and talk to someone as you walk down the street.

© 2024 - My Peace of Health, LLC

Likewise, every lunch date will not lead to some new life-altering friendship – and that's OK! Don't seek out lots of people, nor should you measure your success by quantity. Quality is what you seek. Find the ones that feel genuine and meaningful to you. Let the rest go.

Now it's time for the good parts – and if you weren't already aware, knowing people and having friends can be good for you! Specifically, people with tight social bonds experience lower levels of stress and have improved mental health and a greater likelihood of longevity. Who wouldn't want someone to laugh with, to talk to, or to share the worst and best moments in life with?

In this beautiful season of making friends and building relationships, remember that prayer: 'You did not make us to be alone, but to live in community with others.' As you make friends or remember those loved ones, you are living your way into God's plan. As you have been enriched by those who have walked with you through faith, remember to bless those along the way. Call someone you've lost touch with, touch base with a friend, make a new friend, or celebrate those you 'found' already. Give thanks for God's gift of community so that it can bless your life in many good ways today!

I went online scrolling through Facebook Marketplace looking for some housewares. Lo and behold, some lady posted these adorable, woven baskets, with which I start chatting, and it turns out she's not just any seller, she's a pastor with a side hustle teaching public speaking.

Of course, this encourages me to come too, and I became part of her circle of women looking to find their voice. True, I was initially jittery and unsure of my skills. These ladies were pros. I had some things to learn. But the fear of appearing foolish waned in the face of my hunger to improve. And I did learn a great deal.

But even more than that, there was a sense of community where I could personally question everything, fall, blindly stumble, and still be 100 percent embraced. Where they'd pick me up when I tumbled, and root me on when I soared. A personal cheer squad of friends.

© 2024 - My Peace of Health, LLC

And best of all: through all those peaks and valleys, I learned it's okay to suck – that's where the magic happens. And, by having that community behind me, I was able to step into my own as a coach and mentor.

But you know what? I still consider some of them from this group my friends, years later. I miss those bonding days and make a point of catching up whenever I can. Finding your tribe isn't just about learning a skill – it's about forming lifelong friendships and sticking together through thick and thin.

Let's unpack these dynamics of relationships and how they affect our happiness at the micro and macro levels. Brace yourself, because this is going to get nerdy and awesome at the same time because there is so much fascinating research and expert opinion out there.

Research Findings:

The science is getting clearer. New analyses are making it abundantly clear: our social connections have a direct impact on both our mental and physical health. In one meta-analysis – a study of studies – in the Journal of Health and Social Behavior, researchers found that people with good social support have about a 50 percent greater chance of survival than those who braved life alone. We are in this together.

Dr. Neil Nedley, a renowned physician and author, brings a unique perspective to the table when it comes to the intersection of relationships and well-being. As the founder of the Nedley Depression and Anxiety Recovery Program, he has delved into the intricate links between mental health and various aspects of life, including relationships.

"Good relationships with family and friends are critical for a person's mental and emotional wellness," says Dr Nedley, whose research and clinical experience confirmed that healthy personal connections can be a vital antidote to suffering caused by depression, anxiety, and other disorders. He's a firm believer in the power of healing 'connection' – through the acceptance, support, and validation of loved ones who truly care for your wellbeing, and that acceptance strengthens one's sense of identity and worth.

© 2024 - My Peace of Health, LLC

Furthermore, he emphasizes the need to focus on relational conflicts and stressors as a 'holistic' form of mental health care. Working with both patients and their loved ones to develop effective communication, empathy, and conflict resolution skills helps to improve peoples' overall emotional well-being and create supportive social systems.

In other words, Dr. Nedley is asking us to recognize the fundamental influence of relationships on mental health and to prioritize consoling relationships as an integral part of a healthful life – one that, as this story about an alternative approach to therapy shows, can be intimately tied to our human relationships.

With that, we bring our chapter on how to develop robust relationships to a close. It's worth underlining the vital part that the quality of our relationships plays in wellness and flourishing – in how our lives feel and go, from intimate personal bonds to profound connections. Our relationships with parents and romantic partners can be sources of pleasure and suffering, of joy and distress. Friendships enrich our lives, and their loss can be painful, even devastating. As a society, we have begun to recognize that our relational lives are central to achieving health and happiness.

In this chapter, we've looked up and down and all around at the different kinds of relationships, from the all-over-the-place experience of marriage and partnership to the amazement and angst of parenting, to the power and peril of developing friends and even community, and all the while, looked at the research evidence, the wisdom of the experts and some practical tools for making relationships better, for getting on better together, for using conflict statements and connection statements, to enrich our interactions and our lives.

When it comes to navigating the intricacies of intimacy, the truth is that all relationships are so very different. Some may be richer in certain aspects, while poorer in others, but the key seems to be to stay committed to the connections you have, with each relationship, and to keep trying to find ways to make them better, sharing our power with our friends and loved ones, and remembering their valuable contributions, while also remembering to take care of and prioritize ourselves as individuals too.

© 2024 - My Peace of Health, LLC

Discussion Questions

1. Reflecting on your experiences, how have relationships influenced your overall wellness and happiness?

2. How do you cultivate connections with others? What tools and rituals do you draw on to enable connection in your relationships?

3. Talk about a difficult experience in a relationship and how you got through it. What did you take from that?

© 2024 - My Peace of Health, LLC

4. Why is communicating with someone you care about important?
    How do you normally communicate during conflicts and
    disagreements?

5. Think of a time when you were supported by your community or
    friends – how did your health improve?

© 2024 - My Peace of Health, LLC

© 2024 - My Peace of Health, LLC

© 2024 - My Peace of Health, LLC

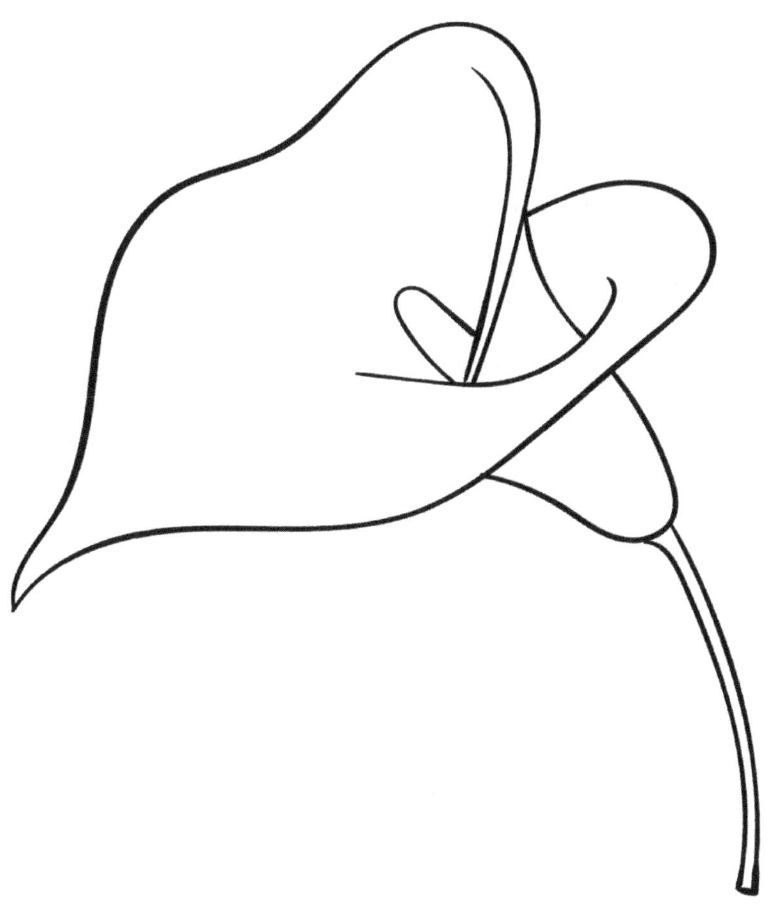

© 2024 - My Peace of Health, LLC

© 2024 - My Peace of Health, LLC

Chapter 4

Thriving Through Transitions

Shifting from one career to another comes with uncertain ups and downs, fear, and new challenges. I'll take you back to February 2008 when I was an LPN working in pediatrics in Chicago. I was all set to begin climbing the career ladder. Then… everything changed!

It was Black History Month at my children's school. My eldest son (aged six at the time) stood at the mic, without my knowledge, with his eyes on fire, and recited Langston Hughes' I, Too from memory. You see, I should tell you something about my little boy. He was quiet and shy, so seeing him on stage felt like a ton of bricks.

And the cherry on top? My daughter was also in the program – but while her peers were dancing to the African number, mine was marching to her beat in silent circles with a big grin on her face. Pure, unrestrained joy; the moment that said, in essence, 'Hey, how much do you know about what's going on at your kid's school, and how special each of their personalities is?'

Fast forward to a baby on the way and a burning desire for more flexibility to be there for my family. Cue the transition to full-time stay-at-home momma mode—a move that rocked my world and had me questioning my sense of purpose outside the workplace. But let me tell you, it was a journey filled with growth, challenges, and lots of love.

Now add on a move across the country, from Chicago to Arizona, another move to Florida hop, skip, and a jump away, where my husband ran into some challenges with his new gig (supposed to be the most magical place on Earth – or at least in Florida), my health continued to deteriorate, and my marriage was just a hot mess. Instability and uncertainty at their finest. But in chaos, I made the bold move to homeschool my crew of four, seeking stability and connection during the storm.

© 2024 - My Peace of Health, LLC

Homeschooling? I'm not denying that, when we first decided to do it, it felt like leaping off a cliff without a parachute. But also, I'm not sure there was any move we could have made back then that could have preserved our family life – and our sanity – to the extent that this did, especially five years later when the pandemic introduced the rest of the world to the idea of education at home. Homeschooling then became a way to bring them some kind of normalcy and routine amid chaos, a way to get the best of them and connect with them in the deepest possible way, because they needed it so badly, just like me.

Through all this change, I've learned that it's hard but that it can be a gift and even offer growth, that stepping out of the comfortable and familiar and taking a big step into the unknown often awakens things inside of us – even if it feels bumpy and winding.

Let's consider the ultimate example of someone negotiating his way through life's transitions: Jesus of Nazareth. He faced the climb of his life — mountain-scaling the Mount Everest of transitions. And when, at the other side of his transition — death on the cross — his disciples found themselves facing the realities of 'after Jesus', they were fearful, confused, and doubtful. Who wouldn't be? Just think about the situation — an unbelievably unjust and ugly end to a life that had profound meaning for them, for his mother Mary, and for everyone who had ever experienced the love of this remarkable man.

But the thing is, just like Joseph's story didn't end in the pit or the prison, and neither did Jesus's. His death was only the start of something more, the ultimate story of the underdog. His resurrection opened the door for us to experience a new life, even in our graveyards.

My life is currently in a bit of a transition. Today my own nest has taken a major step towards emptying. My older kids are flapping their wings and preparing to fly into adulthood. One even joined the military. I am proud of them. And anxious. And a little bit weepy.

It's like there's this whirlwind of emotions swirling around, and you're just trying to keep your balance amidst the chaos. This parenting gig is a beautiful one, but man, nobody hands you a guidebook for when your

© 2024 - My Peace of Health, LLC

little chicks start leaving the nest. It's like, "Wait, wasn't I just changing diapers and singing lullabies yesterday?"

Even though there's no manual for navigating these transitions, there's something kind of beautiful about it all. It's like this bittersweet symphony of watching your kids grow and flourish, even as your heart aches a little knowing they're spreading their wings and venturing out into the big wide world.

But you know what keeps me moving? Knowing that life's transitions aren't transitions at all but just threads in a tapestry – God's tapestry if you will. I'm praying more, studying scripture more deeply, and trusting that God has this. Like it was for Jesus, the end of our stories may not be the end of our stories at all.

For my sister who is in desperate need of peace amidst life's transitions, let's explore the emotional and psychological dimensions of navigating change. Picture yourself on this wild ride, facing the unknown head-on, with a heart full of courage and a spirit ready to conquer any challenge that comes your way.

Grief

Firstly, there is the grieving process. The loss of a significant milestone (move to another city or another career or whatever) often brings with it grief about your past, and what you had and no longer have. Feel your grief and sadness about what you lose, but remember that it is part of the passage, the process, and then move on.

Identity

Next is the identity shift. You are closing one chapter in your life for another. Who am I now? Where am I going? What might I become? It can be frightening or exhilarating to find out what you're made of and what's coming up next. But here's the thing: you've got resilience running through your veins. It's that God-given strength to rise out of the ashes, to stand firm when the ground shakes, and to become the woman God created you to be. And the beautiful thing is you're never alone on your journey. Lean into your faith and your community and let the love of

© 2024 - My Peace of Health, LLC

those who are standing with you lift you with their prayers and encouragement.

Not to mention support. Remember all those healthy coping mechanisms you know about? Find yours – journaling, painting, moving– and dive in! They're going to be your life raft as you swing from 'up' to 'down' on life's roller coaster.

But the real tea is transitions aren't endings, they're beginnings. Your chance to get started, to grow, to evolve, to chase after your deepest, truest, most wildest dreams. So go grab life by its horns! Get in where you fit in! You are right where you oughta be: because you are in the palm of God's hand.

I'd like to introduce you to my friend Lauren, whose story – of loss and renewal – so clearly illustrates the healing benefits of an emphasis on physical wellness in difficult times.

Now, Lauren's world was turned upside down. In a matter of moments, her 12-year marriage ended in a tragic car accident and she was overwhelmed with grief at losing the man she loved. At 42 years of age, Lauren was gripped by a sense of hopelessness and shattered by the realization that life is a fleeting moment. Alone and in turmoil, she turned to me for help.

Since Lauren loved working out and often turned to physical activity as a means of dealing with distress, I requested that she give exercise a chance to accompany her along her grief journey. Neither of us believed a morning workout would erase any of her painful memories or heal all the emotional pain she carried. But we both hoped a focus on physical health would stand beside her during her most trying times.

The two of us devised a fitness routine that targeted her energy level and inclinations, alternating between cardio, weight-bearing, and walking, but our weekly sessions – more than just an exercise program – evolved into an opportunity for Lauren to vent, to grieve and, most importantly, to find a crack or two in which to reach out and get a handle on the pain.

© 2024 - My Peace of Health, LLC

Gradually, in those months as I continued to watch, it was like I was seeing a completely different person. In the routine of getting healthy, she was getting strong, and not just physically. The endorphins were giving her joy and peace; the physical effort was giving her mental resilience. Her heart began to feel more light.

Further, perhaps most importantly, the sense of camaraderie and support she found in our fitness sessions and in her grit and determination to show up for them, served as a kind of support – she's not doing this alone – as she navigated through her grief. Lauren gave a fight both on and off the floor, and her fight through the darkest of days has made me a better person by showing me the true transformative power of physical health.

To this day, She tries to hold to those virtues by continuing to live her life with courage, embracing each moment as a gift. She says: 'Not a day goes by when I don't miss Mike. The loss is always there. But I learn to live with it and move on so, for the most part, I'm okay.' Fitness has been a wonderful healing balm for navigating life post-loss. Her transformation offers tangible proof that, despite the devastating loss, the light of joy and self-care can once again shine brightly.

Embracing Physical Well-being as a New Beginning:

Keeping ourselves physically well is the biggest transition we should always be making. It sounds like this might be a particularly good time to talk about physical health: transitioning to physical well-being is an essential way that resilience creates space to weather and manage change, and it's also a crucial way of maintaining the strength and vitality of the self as it transitions.

Now the physical: your fitness for the transition. Just as promoting mental fitness is part of survival, so too is attention to physical fitness. We can use natural coping to face the emotional ride of life. When we are going through transitions, to promote our fitness to survive, we must commit to regular and ongoing exercise, good nutrition, and sufficient rest through sleep.

© 2024 - My Peace of Health, LLC

Schedule regular exercise breaks to pep up your energy levels and manage stress. It can be a brisk walk or a workout regimen, but choose an activity of your liking that keeps you fit and active.

Finally, be sure to pay attention to nutrition. If you have the time, meal planning can help ensure (ahead of time) that you fuel your body with healthy foods even if life gets busy. Keeping healthy snack options and pre-made meals on hand can also make it easier to eat nutritiously during hectic days.

And, of course, enough restful sleep. After all, sleep – both in quantity and quality – is necessary for good health. So, be sure to develop a regular bedtime routine and a sleep-friendly environment to ensure sound sleep.

Additionally, practicing relaxation can help with stress management and creates an opportunity to be more grounding and calm during a transition. Self-loving care practices, deep breathing, or journaling are examples – just do whatever feels right for you and find some time each day to practice it.

When you take care of your physical health, you're setting yourself up with the power and strength to move through transitions with poise and vitality. Transitions are not endings but beginnings – an opportunity to embrace the health of your physical body and go after your dreams with abandon, chasing after the Mary we know dreams of righteousness, mercy, and beauty. Embrace this time for your physical health and go after your dreams with gusto because you are in the hands of God.

Holistic Approach to Health

As we dig deeper into the importance of keeping ourselves physically fit during transitions, it's crucial to recognize how our physical, mental, and spiritual well-being are all connected. Taking a holistic approach to our health means we're not just focusing on our bodies, but also on our minds and spirits, especially when life throws us curveballs.

While exercising, eating healthily, and sleeping well, let us also attend to our spiritual well-being. For Christians, that could be taking a few

© 2024 - My Peace of Health, LLC

moments for prayer and meditation upon the Scriptures, or just holding back from the constant talking and praying over our complicated lives and seeking God's presence in our everyday activities. These are also means of finding peace in disquiet.

And while we're at it, let us have fun and enjoy ourselves too! Whether it's going for a walk and immersing ourselves in nature or being mindfully grateful for what we have painting, words, and stories, all these activities can provide meaning and a sense of well-being as well.

Yes, by tending to all aspects of our being – body, mind, and soul – we are better positioned to make it through life's transitions. And remember, you are not alone. God is walking with you every step of the way into every twist and turn of life. Let's walk together in the way of this whole-person health and enter through life's transitions as whole, authentic, knowingly holy people.

Embracing Connection: Nourishing Relationships Amid Transition

But with all the talk of leading healthy lives and practicing self-care, we cannot lose sight of the value of relationships. Although life is a physical, intellectual, and spiritual journey, nourishing our relationships with others is every bit as gratifying and productive as reading a good book or having a good soak in the tub.

Reach Out: Transition can seem more manageable with a hand to hold. Open up your heart and reach out to friends, relatives, or others with whom you feel comfortable sharing emotions. Ask them to celebrate your victories and stand by your side through your disappointments. The human touch is a valuable resource in allowing us to open up.

Celebrate Together: During every phase of life, celebrate milestones together – the big ones and small ones – with your friends and family. Share a meal, offer solace with a kind ear, or throw a party. Celebrate the moments – both great and small – for both are cause for joy.

Lean on Your Faith: They say that life is an up-and-down affair so lean on your faith … Accept that God goes with you through every move, from apartment to house to retirement, and that He will help you find the

© 2024 - My Peace of Health, LLC

right place and calm your heart in the transition. Ask for help from your 'home church' for their prayers and support.

Stay in touch: Make sure you maintain good relationships with those you love and care about, both near and far, by meeting regularly and engaging in quality interactions. Call someone you haven't spoken to in a while. Write a card or letter. Zoom or Skype with friends or family living far away.

Create New Relationships: Seize opportunities to create new relationships and expand your social network, especially when you are experiencing life's disruptions. Join a club, or volunteer at a church or community group where you share an interest or value with others and that will yield new friends and meaningful alliances.

Holding the space that allows us to express our full selves, in the journey towards whole-person health, the most precious gift is our relationships with others. Together, we embrace life's transitions, in a mutuality of resilience, knowing that we have each other's back, know each other more fully, and are loved more completely.

So, how do we cope with life's transitions and emerge even stronger on the other side? Here are some key strategies to help you navigate change, loss, and adversity with peace and resilience:

1. **Acceptance**: Beloved, embrace your reality. Trust in God's plan. Allow yourself to feel your feelings. Know that God holds your tomorrow in His hands.
2. **Seek Support**: Surround yourself with fellow believers who will give you encouragement, support, and advice, and pray with you over the challenging things that come up in life.
3. **Practice Self-Forgiveness:** Be kind to yourself, you're child of God, as God is to you, granting you compassion, forgiveness, and grace. Forgive yourself, and know who God knows you to be.
4. **Find Meaning:** Seek God's purpose in every situation. Even in the darkest moments, His light shines through, revealing lessons to be learned and blessings to be found.

© 2024 - My Peace of Health, LLC

5. **Take Care of Yourself:** Honor the body of the Holy Spirit within you, beloved. Treat your Temple with dignity, nurturing your body, mind, and spirit through practices that honor God's gift of life.
6. **Stay Flexible:** Give up, darling. Give up to God's plans. Trust Him and stay flexible, because God will make all things work together for your good.
7. **Focus on What You Can Control:** Surrender control to the One who holds the universe in His hands, dear one. Trust in God's providence and focus on aligning your will with His divine purpose.
8. **Practice Gratitude:** Thank God for the abundance of His gifts, dear child. Cultivate a grateful heart, for He is good in every way.
9. **Stay Connected to Your Faith**: Draw near to God in prayer and meditation. Anchor your soul in His promises, knowing that He is your rock and your fortress in times of trouble.
10. **Embrace Change as a Growth Opportunity:** Be limited no more, child of God! Imagine change as the gift of growth, and trust that God will guide you towards the path of more faith and fulfillment.

You are deeply loved, cherished, and guided by the hand of God, dear one. Embrace His love, trust in His plan, and walk confidently into the beautiful future He has prepared for you.

© 2024 - My Peace of Health, LLC

Let's dive into some journal prompts designed to help you navigate life's transitions with faith and resilience:

1. **Reflect on a past transition**: I want you to think of a significant transition in your life. What was difficult about that time for you? How did the Lord bring you through? Write it out and let those memories serve as proof of God's faithfulness.

2. **Consider your current transition:** What transition are you walking through? Pause. Check in with your emotions. Fearful? Hoping? Doubting? Tell Jesus. Tell Him all you're feeling. Write it down. Let the peace of God flood over you.

© 2024 - My Peace of Health, LLC

3. **Visualize your dream outcome:** Imagine yourself already on the other side of the transition, walking with Jesus, hand in hand. What does winning look like for you? What does the journey there look like? What steps can you take to get there? Quiet your mind and your heart, dear sister, and give your desires to Him. He will lead the way.

© 2024 - My Peace of Health, LLC

© 2024 - My Peace of Health, LLC

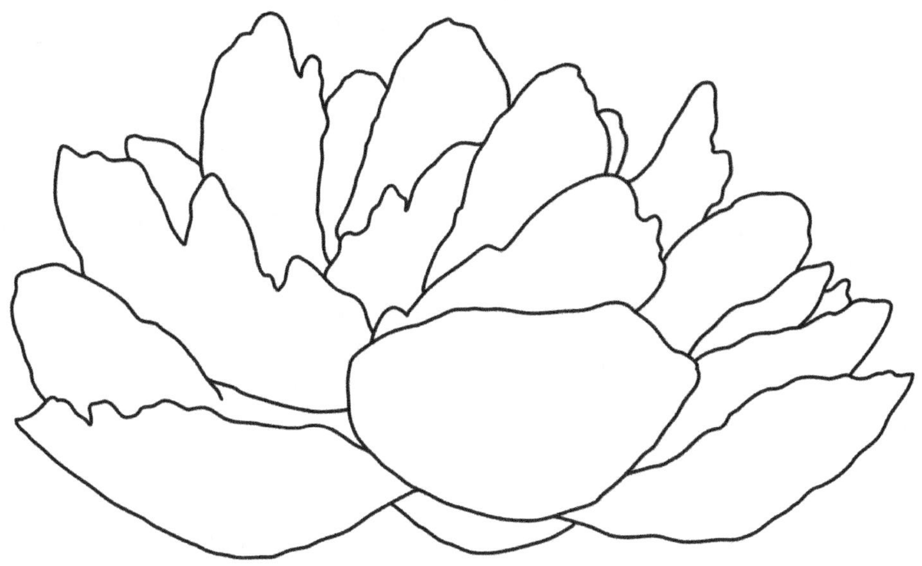

© 2024 - My Peace of Health, LLC

© 2024 - My Peace of Health, LLC

Chapter 5

Balancing Work and Life

Let me tell you about another client/friend, Shevon. Shevon has two small children and works full-time. She is a loving mom and a dedicated employee. But right now she is struggling. She feels overwhelmed and burned out.

She gets up before dawn, makes breakfast, gets her kids dressed, gets them to school and herself to work. From sunup to sundown between meetings, deadlines, and emails she practically flies from one work-related obligation to another, all with her kids' lives on her mind and all the while feeling bad for not spending enough time with them.

She returns in the evening, bone-tired, brain-tired, there are rush-hour dinners and a creeping feeling that she will never again have even a spare minute to work on her ambitions, never mind to have even a private moment with her children.

Shevon's Pain Points:

- Feeling Overwhelmed: Shevon scatters herself at work and home, cracking up and running out of energy.
- Guilt and Worry: Shevon feels guilty about the time she doesn't spend with her kids and worries about them constantly.
- Lack of Personal Time: Her work schedule makes it very difficult for her to find time for herself. Her passions and dreams are difficult to pursue.

Sound familiar? If so, then you've got plenty of company among the women I know. The corporate limbo that Shevon found herself in is the pattern I hear about from most of the women I coach – as well as my friends, family members, and, yes, parts of my own life. The dance-dance of work-family-self.

© 2024 - My Peace of Health, LLC

We call it mom guilt. That feeling that we're not good enough, that we're not doing enough, that we've made the wrong choice, that we put ourselves above our children, etc.

How many times have you felt like this? You love your children, you want what's best, and yet you easily feel guilty – you've gone to the work awards dinner when the school fair is on, you've been out for dinner with friends when you thought you should be at home, enjoying every spare second you could get. It can cast a dark cloud over even your very happiest moments. Mom's guilt is ubiquitous.

Only one thing is for sure: if you have kids– whether it's your first, your fifth, your own, or your step-, adoptive, or foster, your children can trigger the driest, arid, withering feeling in your soul. You question whether you're 'good enough', whether you're 'failing', when the truth is: that you are doing the best you can with what you've got. You are loving them to pieces. You are feeding them. You are showing them the lessons you think they need to learn.

Be ready to feel mom guilt – it will ebb and flow, no question – but don't let it take over. Instead, let the love for your kiddo (and the things you do for and with her/him) take over your thoughts.

And remember you're not alone – mom guilt strikes most of us at some point or another, so share your worries and frustrations with friends and family members, who can remind you of the awesome mom you are.

Sis, I know it's not easy balancing work and family and still keeping your spiritual life up. But don't worry, God has provided us with the power and insight to do so, in peace.

Trust in Divine Timing

Think back to the story of Mary and Martha. In Luke 10:38-42, these two sisters welcome Jesus to their house. One of them (Martha) is bustling around, while the other (Mary) just sits at Jesus' feet with her behind planted on the floor, listening to him speak. Martha is mad, I bet. 'Hey Jesus,' she tells him, 'can you get Mary up off the floor so she can help me around here?' Jesus: 'Martha, Martha…' Yeah, you know the rest.

© 2024 - My Peace of Health, LLC

As Mary did, we need to step back, sit at Jesus' feet, seek God's wisdom, and appreciate God's grace. Don't be scared to leave the activity of making dinner for others. Trust God's timing. And the rest will fall into place. You can bet your bottom dollar on it.

Lean on Your Support System

I'll keep saying this: It was never for us to go it alone. As Ruth did under the care of Naomi (Ruth 1:16-17), we can lean on our support (be it spouse, family, friends, or fellow believers) and share with them our burdens, as well as our joys. We can let them walk with us in prayer and encouragement. Carrying each other's burdens and sharing each other's load, we will find, indeed, that together no load is as heavy as when we go it alone.

Set Healthy Boundaries

Be good to your body, your mind, and your spirit as daughters of the King. Guard your times and places in your work and your personal life to give proper attention to the things of God and the people of God, and to protect yourself from the bombardment of evil in the world. Rest and restore often – in solitude, and like Jesus, in lonely places of prayer. Let God do the work he longs to do for you when you guard your time and energy for Him. He waits to fill your bones with his peace and joy.

Find Joy in the Journey

Meanwhile, sweet sister, never overlook the importance of the journey itself. Believe me, you will want to relish the sweetness of your moments, rejoice at your tiny triumphs, enjoy your children, and give thanks to God for all of His good gifts. Do not forget to celebrate life, to remember that life is a gift, and to glorify God by reflecting his love into the faces of others.

Please surrender your ambitions and plans to the Lord and trust that He shall guide you every moment of your life. When your faith becomes

© 2024 - My Peace of Health, LLC

your guide and you are enveloped in His love, life becomes graceful, peaceful, and joyful.

Setting boundaries, keeping priorities straight, and avoiding burnout.

Now for the big one: boundaries. Boundaries are the guardrails of the highway of life.

What are they, then? Boundaries are about what we place, outside ourselves, that tell others where they can't trespass, to protect ourselves, our energy, and our very sanity. Boundaries are about what's acceptable for us and what isn't. Boundaries are about what others can and cannot do, and how we communicate and express our desire for things to stay within a certain zone. Boundaries are about the no-go zones we create for ourselves in a relationship when it comes to our well-being, to prevent being harassed with stress, overwhelmed, and resentment.

It seems to be an intimidating concept, at first glance, but when we start to think and act in these terms, we'll be more likely to prioritize what matters to us and what doesn't, to say 'no', and to stand up for ourselves.

The thing is, boundaries can come in all kinds of shapes, sizes, and forms. Maybe it's simply saying 'no' to that one more thing at work (whilst you're already working yourself into the ground). Or maybe it's setting some healthy, protective boundaries and making sure you allocate time for what I'd like to call 'womb time' – a sacred 'me' time to help you unwind and recharge every day. Or maybe it's about building and asserting clear boundaries about how you would like to be treated in relationships – whether it be with your spouse, your family, your friends, or even your colleagues.

© 2024 - My Peace of Health, LLC

However, here's the kicker: boundaries aren't just about saying no. They are also about saying yes to you – to you and your needs, wants, and care. They are about making space for the things that get you going, for the things that bring you joy, whether it's finding time for a passion project, for loved ones, or just for a well-deserved self-care session.

So how do you do it? First, it's a matter of getting crystal clear and honest about the things that are most important to you, and the things that are not. And then it's about communicating those limits –, confidently, and with more than just a bit of grace…and without apology.

Remember that boundary setting is the expression of self-love, self-respect, and personal integrity. It is not unkindness or a lack of concern for others. Boundary setting means self-care. It focuses on your rights, your needs, and, most of all, your well-being. It is uncomfortable because it often involves disappointing others, and hovering over the choppy waters of risk and change. But trust me, the sense of peace and freedom on the other side of the shore is worth it.

However, so be it: do it, dear friend – I need you to do it – and do it like the boss you are. Do it because sheer survival – your happiness, sanity, well-being – depends on it.

Managing Priorities

Just so we're clear: you can't do it all, and that's OK. You've considered this before, and you know what you're like when you're at your best. Are you being your best self if you have too little time for your family? For your passions? For just breathing? If you're not clear about your priorities, you might start with your values. What enlivens your heart? What is the highest purpose for your life?

It's the ability to maintain a strong focus on matters of importance in a world full of tumult and noise. It's like conducting an orchestra: all of your responsibilities playing different instruments and making their musical contributions.

© 2024 - My Peace of Health, LLC

So how do you manage priorities? You have to determine what you are called to do, and what your heart likes to do, and then you put the things that you like to do in front of everything else that you do.

The deal is this: you have a limited number of years to live and a limited number of hours every week. So the real question you need to ask yourself is what is it that you value so much that you would spend your precious energy to help make it happen?

Managing priorities is like being a captain of a ship: you set a course and set sail to places you want to arrive. It's a deliberate way of spending your time and using your resources to do more of the things that you like, that matter, or bring you joy.

But let me be honest: managing priorities is not always easy. Life happens. It throws curveballs, chases shiny objects, or pulls you in a hundred different directions.

That's why it helps to have a plan – a roadmap if you will – to stay on track. Maybe that means using a to-do list or a weekly planner to keep you organized and goal-oriented. Or maybe it means giving yourself specific goals and deadlines to keep yourself motivated and accountable.

The truth is, that prioritization is, at base, a matter of living intentionally and purposefully. It's about designing a life – a world – that you value and are passionate about. Then it's all about purposefully acting to bring that world you envisioned into reality.

So go on, pull the reins; and get control of your priorities; your success, your satisfaction, and your happiness are right there waiting for you!

Avoiding Burnout

I'd been homeschooling our four children – grades ranging between kindergarten to seventh grade – for a little over a year and felt myself flailing in a slough of burnout. Every day was a monumental effort to decipher the different curricula and teach the children concurrently. Nothing seemed to click for anyone, and I was ready to quit.

© 2024 - My Peace of Health, LLC

My inability to say no – to learn to set my boundaries – made all of this only worse. I volunteered to teach the church children so my kids would have a rich church experience and also found myself leading our little group in the Adventurer Club, which is the Christian version of scouts. I felt pressure to make our weekly game nights take place at our house (even though I would be so spent).

But, as an introvert, I found that the amount of social interaction depleted me even more than I already felt, and I had no reserves left. I loved my husband and children and friends but I longed for quiet and rest and removed the hustle and bustle of the demands of daily living.

And in the middle of that mess, I felt that something had to give, too. I started to set boundaries and take better care of myself, saying no to commitments that would suck my energy and yes to activities that fed me. Now, with my husband's support and boundless faith, I've been fortunate to regain a measure of control over my time and energy.

This didn't happen overnight, and there were many false starts and setbacks in the process. But with every small step I took, I got a little better aligned and, in time, remembered and recovered a way of living in harmony and balance with myself and with the world around me. Along that path of self-recognition and renewal came the peace and well-being my life had somehow lost.

Burnout? Ain't nobody got time for that! Seriously now… Burn-out… It's like running a car at full speed straight into a wall – not pretty. It's that little monster lurking around the corner, ready to bite you at any moment. Trust me, it's like jumping from thunderstorm drips, but with the right knowledge, you can stay dry and keep on moving! It's that feeling of fatigue, overwhelm, and complete depletion you get after pushing yourself too hard for too long. It's your body's way of shouting to you, of saying: 'You are doing too much! Slow down!'

And burn-out is different than exhaustion. It's more of an emotional and mental depletion, too. To be bone tired and burnt out means that you are running on fumes, that you have nothing left to give.

© 2024 - My Peace of Health, LLC

So what can you do to prevent burnout, then? Well, it's all about awareness, of being aware of your limits and waking up before you're too deep into something before you've been burnt out for too long. So you know when to stop – when to say enough is enough. And so, are you grumpy and irritable every day? Can you no longer pay attention to what you're doing? Whatever it is that signals to you that you are overdoing it, listen to yourself and listen to your body.

And the main thing is balance – of work and me-time, of rest and activity, of what you give out to others and of what you receive in return. Of what time you give yourself to the things you enjoy, that are meaningful to you – be it to connect with family and friends, or of pursuing your hobbies or interest, or of giving yourself the time to breathe and just be…So, do me a favor, my friend. Put your health first, and make avoiding "burnout" your number-one priority. You don't want to burn your health, do you? You don't want to be unhappy and you don't want to lose your mind?

Avoiding burnout is crucial for maintaining your well-being and productivity. It's like taking care of a delicate flower—you need to nurture yourself to stay vibrant and healthy. Here are some tips to help you steer clear of burnout:

- **Self-Care Is Important**: Give yourself some time to replenish your batteries (eg, read a book, go for a walk, do some hobbies) because as I've said before, you cannot pour from an empty cup.
- **Set Boundaries**: Say 'no' to anything extra that will pull you too thin. Your time and energy are valuable; guard them like a hawk.
- **Delegate When Possible:** If you can get help from others, feel free to do so! Don't beat yourself up for not being able to do it all.
- **Sleep**: Get enough! Nothing can restore the body and brain like adequate restorative sleep.
- **Stay Active:** Regular exercise promotes mental health. Get as active as you can, finding activities that you enjoy.
- **Connect with Others:** Don't underestimate the restorative power of social connections. Whether it's a loved one or joining a club or support group, stay connected to others.

© 2024 - My Peace of Health, LLC

- **Seek Professional Help If Needed**: If you already feel overwhelmed, please seek help from a mental health professional and get the support and tools you need.

Remember, avoiding burnout means taking steps to care for yourself daily and avoid overextending. When you self-care and set boundaries on your work, you'll be able to avoid burnout and live a full, happy life!

Biblical Support and Coaching Advice

With this in mind, let's consider some biblical backing and coaching to get you on your way:

1. **Believe in God's Plan:** 'Commit your works to the Lord, and your plans will be established' (Proverbs 16:3). Trust God to have a wonderful plan for your life, and that He will lead you at each step.
2. **Stay grounded:** Philippians 4:13: I can do all things through Him who strengthens me. Lean on your faith as you run after your dreams because God is with you.
3. **Get wise counsel:** Proverbs 15:22: 'Plans fail for lack of counsel, but with many advisers they succeed.' Who is your wise counsel — a wise mentor, coach, or friend?

As you pursue your passions, goals, and dreams with peace and intentionality, remember that you are capable of achieving greatness. With faith as your guide and purpose as your compass, there's no limit to what you can accomplish.

So go ahead, dream big my friend, and pursue those dreams with all your heart. You'll find your purpose when you finally open your arms to it.

© 2024 - My Peace of Health, LLC

Discussion Questions

1. How am I defining success in my work and personal life right now? Are these definitions reflective of my values and priorities?

2. What are the biggest stressors for me in my life right now? How are these stressors affecting my ability to balance my work life and personal life?

3. If I take a look at my average weekday and weekend routine, how am I spending my time on work tasks, personal tasks, leisure and exercise, or self-care activities?

© 2024 - My Peace of Health, LLC

4. What are some activities or tasks that make me feel more
    energized and joyful? How can I spend more time doing these
    activities?

5. What are some activities or tasks that make me feel more
    drained and contribute to my stress and burnout? How can I do
    less of these activities or delegate them to others?

© 2024 - My Peace of Health, LLC

© 2024 - My Peace of Health, LLC

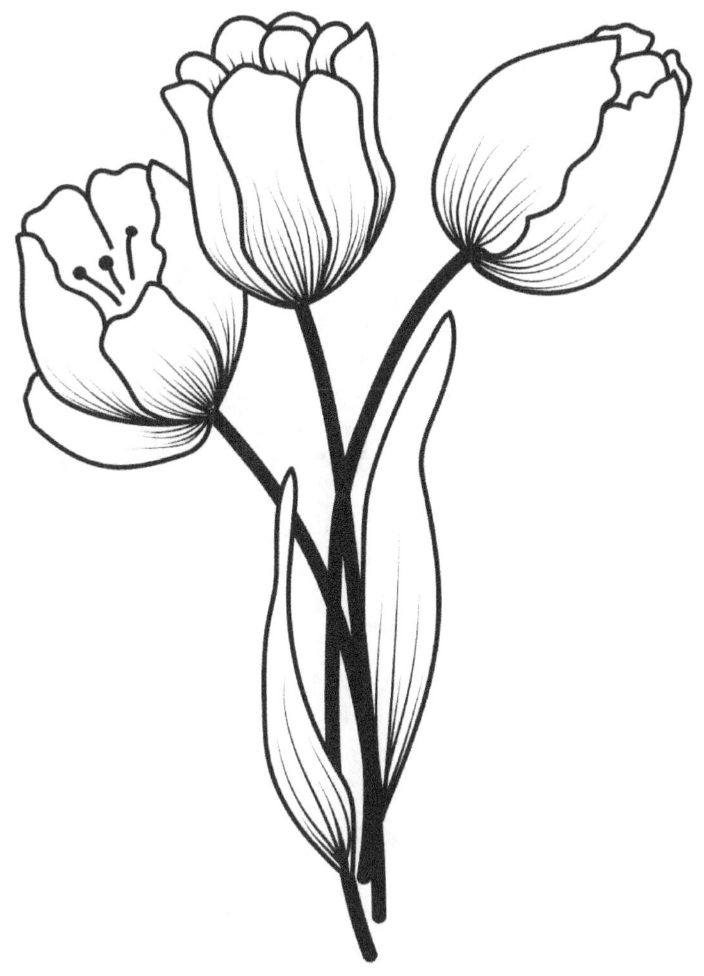

© 2024 - My Peace of Health, LLC

© 2024 - My Peace of Health, LLC

Chapter 6

Cultivating Family Spirituality

Joshua. He was no ordinary Joe. He was a leader. He was a warrior. And, most importantly, he was a loving and loyal husband and father. Life wasn't always easy – it could be painful, it could wander down some dark roads leading him to question his faith, and it could lead him to fear. Whatever the heck he went through, he never stopped believing in God.

Through his weeping, Joshua declared: 'But as for me and my house, we will serve the Lord.' Ripping at the air was not just a statement of intention; it was a call to war, a prayer, and an appeal for solidarity, that they serve the Lord.

And what did you know? It wasn't just a passive response from his family: they were there too, with hearts ready, and full of love and commitment, and they joined him in public worship, in prayer, in the assurance that God had become their rock, their place of safety, their all.

From that day forward, their home became a sanctuary—a spot where God's presence was felt in every nook and cranny, in every chat, in every moment of quiet reflection. They didn't just gather together out of duty—they did it because they couldn't get enough of honoring the One who'd been their constant companion through it all.

And so in the end, they sang their songs at the altar, raising their voices in praise and proclaiming their collective peace and resting in God's infinite, eternal love.

What's the moral of the story? That's easy: it is about love, not ritualism. It's about a guy who wanted his family to know the peace and wellness that he'd found in his relationship with God. It's about a family that said, "Heck yeah, we're all in this together – let's walk with God now and forever."

© 2024 - My Peace of Health, LLC

Building a peaceful home filled with prayer, worship, and spiritual connection.

Okay everyone, here's how to get your home ready to love and be loved in. Let's make this a space that not only feels good but oozes calm and kindness in equal measure. Ready to sprinkle your home with grace and make your nest the comfiest of sanctuaries? Let's start.

So how can we cultivate a more peaceful home? The beauty all happens in the preparation. It's about nurturing the soil so sharing, respect and understanding can flourish. Imagine seeds of caring sown in the soil of your home and blossoming into a garden of peace.

However, life is unpredictable and people get upset and misinterpret. Fear not, because you can find ways to de-escalate tension and make peace at home.

But how do you get there? By starting wherever you are, and leading the way with your example. Showing up with patience and grace when the going gets hard. Take a moment to say a quiet prayer before you respond to a challenging situation. Listening to the various characters in your family who want to share their thoughts. Offering a word of encouragement when someone you love is feeling stressed.

Finally, make room for quietness — both physically and emotionally. Perhaps it's providing a corner with soft pillows and warm blankets, where children and guests can retreat when they need downtime and space to pray and restore their spirits. Or perhaps it's integrating periods of prayer and meditation into the flow of the home, stopping to root yourself in the living presence of God, and finding your direction in Him.

And finally, don't forget to enjoy the quieter moments of peace and harmony as and when they come along. Whether it's a big hug, a shared joke or simply a few minutes spent with eyes locked, pause to give thanks for the small mercies of life.

So, as you sprinkle a little grace and gratitude around your home, may you find joy, connection, and all the warm fuzzies with your loved ones.

© 2024 - My Peace of Health, LLC

May your home be a place of refuge and renewal, where God's love and presence are felt in every corner.

Embracing Prayer

The wonderful world of prayer—it's like having a heart-to-heart chat with the most important person in your life, except that person happens to be the Creator of the universe! How cool is that?

Prayer then, is your direct line to God, the place where you pour out your feelings, your fears, your plans, and your hopes. But it's also a wonderful way to bond with your parents and siblings, to get closer to one another and to God too.

Picture this: it's time for dinner, and you've pulled up chairs around the table. Before you and your family sink your teeth into that veggie pot pie you worked so hard on, you reach out to say the prayer of thanks. A second later, you're both holding hands, and dinner is off to a good, grateful start.

Or this: it's bedtime, and you put your little ones to bed. You sit next to them to say some prayers and ask them to think about what they might want to ask God for or to express thankfulness to Him for. Maybe they thank Him for the day they had at the park and wish God would keep Grandma well who might be under the weather. This moment of sweet communion fills your heart with warmth.

But prayer is not confined to mealtimes and nighttimes. It is for when you are worried and fearful, and want an extra dose of calm and assurance. It is for when you are celebrating a happy event or enjoying a triumph, and want to express thanks to the One who makes it all possible. And it is for when you are walking through valleys of darkness or mountains of difficulty, hoping that God will shine a ray of light on your path ahead.

But what does it look like to embrace prayer as a family? I guess it all boils down to making it an everyday habit – praying grace over your meals, praying with your children before they go to bed, and having a prayer time as a family every morning. Find a time and a place that

© 2024 - My Peace of Health, LLC

works well for you, and make it a sacred moment that you can look forward to each day.

Next, get creative with your prayers! Encourage each family member to share their thoughts, feelings, and intentions with the group. Maybe one day you sing your prayers, and the next day you draw them. The sky's the limit—just let your imagination run wild!

And always, remember that prayer is a road, not a roof; we are praying to a God who is constantly moving us, ever more loving, ever more gentle, ever more present, as we pray together, one prayer at a time. So, be patient with yourselves, and with one another; God is listening, God is loving, God is ready – right where we are.

And as you learn to pray as a family, may you grow closer in love than ever before, may you experience peace and joy in a way you never have before, and may you invoke the presence of God in your midst as a source of love and grace for all who are seeking.

Cultivating Worship

But what is worship, exactly? It's the chance to pray, sing, or pen a private note to God from your heart and soul. This might mean singing your favorite hymns in the sanctuary, strumming your guitar in your living room, or taking in the sights and sounds of God's rainfall as you lift your arms and dance in the puddles.

The point is, that worship isn't just for a weekly service – it is to be lived every hour of every day. It's about doing everything as a sweet-smelling sacrifice to God. Your every thought, word, and deed can be an act of worship. And they can be offered up to God in every moment, whether you are washing dishes or driving to work, visiting with friends or family … you get the idea.

What then is worshipful living? The very first thing is being able to provide some space for the soul and the calendar. Learn to leave yourself some minutes in the day to be spent with God in prayer and meditation, in contemplation. When, in the morning? When the rest of

© 2024 - My Peace of Health, LLC

the earth has just begun to stir and awaken? And at night, when it has grown quiet and still?

Finally, go creative. Worship does not 'look' like anything, or 'sound' like anything, or 'be' anything. Worship does not have to involve clapping, or having to do something, singing, doing drama, painting or poetry, or anything else. All the things you do to God to express your love – the things that communicate to your heart that you are near to God, that you are pouring out. Sing if you like; teach if you like; paint if you like; write if you like; pray if you like. Be a mess. You do not have to worry about messing up, that God loves the right and hates the wrong, that he cares if you do it or get it right or wrong – see, God, is not scared of your mess, he is scared of you pretending to have a tidy heart, being shiny and right and 'on point'. He wants you to show up messy because only you show up this way, only you worship him in this way.

And last, remember that worship is a journey, not a place. It does indeed take you somewhere – closer to God, and more closely connected with others – but this happens prayer by prayer, moment by moment, step by step. So, be patient with yourself, and with God. He isn't going anywhere; he's right there with you, leading you, loving you, and rooting for you the whole way.

May you know more communion, more delight, and more peace, than ever before: as you taste a new understanding of what worship is, and your heart be filled more and more fully with great love and gratitude to the One who loves you with a love that lasts forever.

Passing down our beliefs and values to the next generation.

I was also fortunate to have heard, so many times, the stories of faith and devotion that passed from one generation of our family to another. My grandmother used to sit me down with our family album and walk me through the history of our family's faith, and how we came to know Jesus through my great-grandmother.

She would tell us stories about my widowed great-grandmother, who had no money, and who found everything she needed in Jesus. She would speak of her church that leaked in the rain, and the tent meetings where

© 2024 - My Peace of Health, LLC

souls were saved. The details of her life, and her faith in our church and its ministry, dripped with her love.

It was more than stories: they were living evidence of the power of faith and the inherent rewards of living one's life serving others. My grandmother would speak fondly of stories of my great-grandmother working her fingers to the bone.

And those stories didn't end there: our matriarch – my grandmother, who died a few years ago – took up the mantle and served in the same spirit and manner: stories I now recount to my children: how she was the first to the church; how she came early, ready to set up for the day's events; and when the morning services were over, how she was the last to leave church, ensuring that everything was in order and people were taken care of. She served every weekend, making food to feed the homeless and cutting felts for Sabbath school lesson outlines.

Her life was a living expression of God's love and grace. It gave the Holy Spirit space to spread, and to me, it represented a way of living out one's faith, in whatever we do, for the honor and glory of God. After listening to all her stories and witnessing her faith in action, I reconfirmed my desire to serve wholeheartedly, to love generously, and to live for God.

Because of them, I am who I am. Because of them, I do what I do. Because of them, I have a profound sense of purpose; I desire to serve others as a means of giving and receiving love and compassion. And because of them, I see just how much influence one life who committed her life to faith and service can have on so many others.

That's the effect of passing on spiritual values and traditions: it's about identity, purpose, and meaning, not merely about having a set of rules or beliefs.

This brings me to the question of how we pass on these spiritual stories and traditions to our children. I believe it happens through stories – our own stories of faith and experience, of our meetings with God, of how He has shaped our lives. Every day of our lives should be marked by family devotion and conversation. Meals, bedtime, work, school, play, and

© 2024 - My Peace of Health, LLC

vacation – never a dull moment is missed to gather the little ones around you to pass on a word of advice or wisdom, an insight into our faith.

We've got to not just talk the talk, but also walk the walk – and the best walk to model for our children is one that carries the presence of Jesus: setting aside time for quiet moments with God; praying with and for our kids; regularly engaging in corporate worship; lovingly but humbly confronting our children when they sin; nurturing friendships with those who build us up in the Lord; volunteering at our local shelter; bringing dinner to our friend who just lost her job; loving those who are different than us.

And then there are traditions – the rituals of living that bind us together in families and communities: the ways we eat together at Christmas, the calendars of festivals that mark the passing of the seasons, and the rites of passage that mark our milestones.

And yet: the passing on of spiritual values and practices is not a single moment, but a process, a commitment to practicing throughout life, to maintaining faith – in God and with each other.

In the meantime, don't forget you are not alone. You are standing upon the shoulders of a faith ancestry populated by those who have gone before you, whose stories, traditions, and ideals have made you the person you are today. Their hopes for a better tomorrow will live on through you as you then carry them forward to the next generation. May you approach that journey with love, compassion, and deep gratitude for the gift of faith.

Passing down spiritual values and traditions is a worthwhile, beautiful process that requires intentionality, love, and attention. Here is a list of actions to help you accomplish that:

1. **Live Out Your Faith:** Demonstrate your spiritual beliefs throughout your life rather than just verbalizing them. Your actions should reflect what you feel and believe. Assume a spirit of love, kindness, and compassion.

© 2024 - My Peace of Health, LLC

2. **Share Your Story:** This is where you open up and share with your family what your personal faith journey has been like. Story after story about life, faith, struggles, and unique experiences.
3. **Teach Through Traditions:** Integrate spiritual disciplines and traditions into your family's schedule. Pray before meals. Read religious texts. Keep the Sabbath. Celebrate holidays and religious festivals. Compose rituals to reflect and reinforce your spiritual commitments.
4. **Encourage Dialogue:** The home is the ideal place to form a family culture where exploring questions of faith and service are part of daily living. As much as possible, let your children come to you with their questions and struggles as they naturally arise. Let them explore faith and service without fear of being rebuked. Engage in thoughtful conversations when they have the desire to, providing guidance and support when appropriate.
5. **Involve Children:** Help children engage in meaningful activities and discussions regarding spiritual matters in a manner and at a level commensurate with their age; provide them the opportunity to express their questions, views, and feelings; invite them to participate in family rituals and ceremonies.

Practice these steps and see yourself taking part in the ongoing process of passing on spiritual values and traditions that can sustain faith and love as a new generation shapes the future.

Physical Health

Overall, while this chapter focuses on the topic of family spirituality, the practices, and principles highlighted can support holistic health and wellness by fostering emotional, mental, spiritual, and (ultimately) physical health dimensions for the family.

Let's incorporate elements related to physical health into the discussion:

1. Creating a peaceful home space enhances physical well-being. A home environment should also promote physical health. A clutter-free home and well-kept living space are safer, reducing

© 2024 - My Peace of Health, LLC

risks of accidents or injuries, especially for young children and elderly family members.

2. The chapter makes mention of prayer and worship, but it is important to promote physical activity as part of the family routine to promote healthy behavior. Going on walks as a family or biking and playing sports together are great ways to support this initiative. Physical exercise improves not only one's physical health but also our family relationships as we create positive shared memories while enjoying a healthy and happy life.

3. Encouraging families to introduce more nutritious meals and snacks while cooking and eating together can become organized habits and foster healthier nutrition. Likewise, teaching families to slow down their eating regimens and engage in mindful eating can bolster emotional well-being.

4. Keeping oneself outdoors connected to nature is crucial for physical well-being. Promoting outdoor activities such as gardening, hiking or nature visits enhances the physical workout, reduces stress, and prepares the whole family as far as physical fitness is concerned.

With the integration of these physical health aspects into family life along with spiritual practices, families can offer dimensions of well-being and make room for every member to have good physical, emotional, mental, and spiritual health.

Turning to Scripture for Guidance

Jesus, in the wilderness, fasting for 40 days and nights — his rite of passage and ultimate test of resolve. He's stripped bare, pitted against the world, confronting temptation.

Then, boom! the devil appears, whispering power and glory… the whole package. But Jesus wanted none of it. He hit right back with Scripture, defusing every one of the evil one's schemes.

It's at this moment, Satan tried to twist the Bible to trip Jesus up, but Jesus turned the tables on him with: 'Man shall not live by bread alone, but by every word that comes from the mouth of God' (Matthew 4:4).

© 2024 - My Peace of Health, LLC

And on and on. Every time Satan tried something to trip Him up, Jesus decks him with another verse. 'Don't you put the Lord your God to the test' (Matthew 4:7). 'Get out of here, Satan! For it is written: 'Worship the Lord your God…'' (Matthew 4:10).

It's not just that Jesus is flaunting His knowledge of the Scriptures. It's that He's saying: 'Here's how to deal with temptation when I am putting you under pressure.' It's: 'When life is wearing you down, cling to God's Word as if you need it to live.'

So, when you face unexpected circumstances in life and find yourself unsure of what to do, there is an old and faithful travel companion… you can turn to Scripture. It is your roadmap and guidebook. You can rest assured that it is filled with keys that can unlock the meaning of a life well-lived.

Picture having a cup of tea with a trusted friend who understands the nuances of life as well as anyone. This is what it is like to engage with Scripture: sitting down with the Author of life Himself and learning how to live each day thoughtfully and well from every word.

You can find stories of victory, triumph, quarrels, forgiveness, heroism, horror, and abhorrence in between these holy pages. These Bible stories are meant for both lion and lamb, for you and me. They are there for the discovering and the use, for shaping our own everyday lives.

Whether you're facing big decisions or everyday challenges, Scripture has something to say. It's like having a wise friend whispering in your ear, offering gentle nudges and sage advice to help you navigate life's ups and downs.

When you need encouragement in a tough decision or support for everyday struggles, there's a verse for that. Scripture is like a best friend on your shoulder, gently nudging you or whispering words of wisdom.

© 2024 - My Peace of Health, LLC

Discussion Questions

1. Describe a childhood religious or worldview experience or memory that helped solidify a sense of family connectedness. How did that help to deepen your perspective on family spirituality?

2. What do you already do regularly to encourage a home that supports peace and spirituality? Which of the ideas or practices from this chapter would you like to incorporate into your family life?

© 2024 - My Peace of Health, LLC

3. Think about a time when prayer was central to your family's experience of a challenge or loss. How did prayer help you negotiate that experience? What have you learned from that experience?

4. Can you describe the role that worship plays in your family life? What are the worship practices that you currently employ in your routine family life, and what do you think are the benefits that have resulted from practicing worship at home?

5. Share a spiritual tradition or ritual that is meaningful to your family. What does this tradition mean to you, and how has it helped your family bind together spiritually?

© 2024 - My Peace of Health, LLC

© 2024 - My Peace of Health, LLC

© 2024 - My Peace of Health, LLC

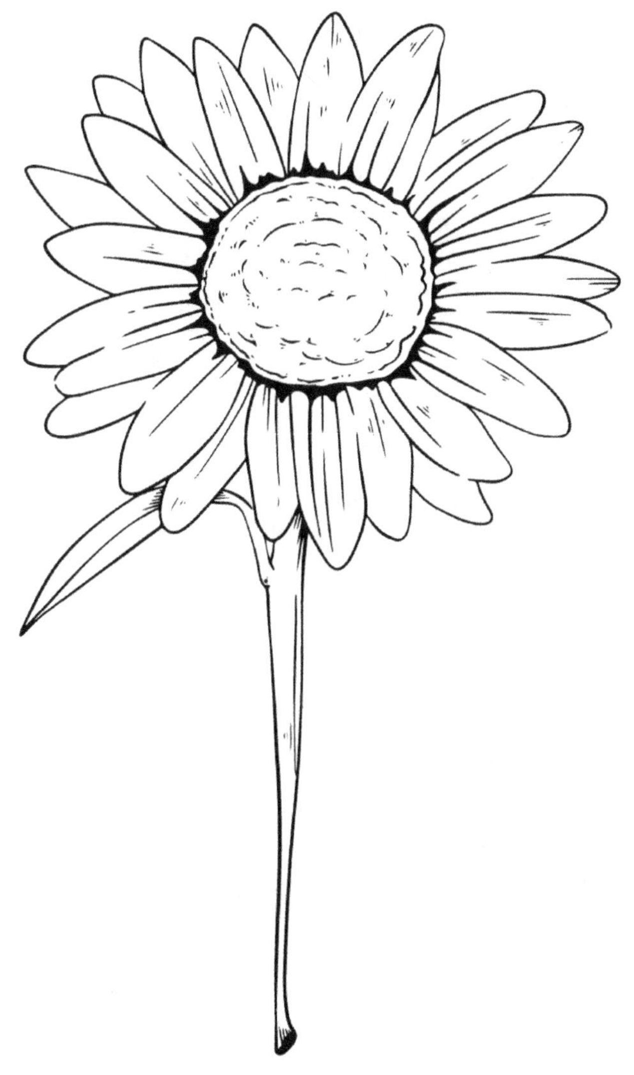

© 2024 - My Peace of Health, LLC

© 2024 - My Peace of Health, LLC

Chapter 7

Creating Peaceful Moments

We wanted to get away from it all for the weekend; we were spending too many hours in the suburbs dragging the children from one activity to another, always on the go. So this weekend's church event, set in the countryside, promised quiet. Such blessings for our souls! We were far from all twitching suburban tensions. We were deeper in the countryside than we normally went. The air was fresher, the reality was slow-paced, and the rhythm more even.

The second we drove in, we saw cabins and green fields and peace. It became a beautiful campsite church with light pouring in and birds singing—pure peace.

The weekend offered opportunities to attend worship services, complete a scavenger hunt, and eat meals with friends, some familiar and some new, in between the deep dives. It was a vacation to refill, replenish, and re-engage in one's faith within a quiet, tranquil environment.

But, as we drove back to the city after our break, the relief of it all turned to shock. The easy quiet of the countryside receded into noise, roadworks, and honking horns. An onslaught, after the bubble-wrapped weekend we'd just enjoyed.

Yet, amid the noise pollution, we held onto the memories of our getaway—the moments of peace, the sense of community, and the spiritual insights gained. As we returned home, we made a pact to seek out tranquility and connection in our everyday lives, no matter how crazy the world around us got.

Appreciate the small things, spending time on the pleasant things in life, creating small memories? Yes, of course. The small things: sitting by a quiet lake, reading by candlelight, and all the other simple pleasures – and that's what I mean when I talk about the quiet things.

© 2024 - My Peace of Health, LLC

Perhaps we should take some pages from the Book of Elijah (you might recall him: he also hung out on Mount Horeb). During great violence and commotion, he did not hear God's voice in the wind, nor in earthquakes and fires, but in a 'still small voice'. Against this deep background noise, he was able to find clarity. Perhaps we too can find clarity – amid the violence and clamor of our lives. All we have to do is listen.

Mental health professionals often highlight the need for a sense of serenity and they might expand on this as follows.

Stress Reduction: Incorporating quiet moments of peace and calm can help lower the physiological harm that can come from chronic stress to our overall mental and physical well-being. Dealing with stressors in our lives makes having moments of calm that much more effective.

Creating a relaxing environment: By finding activities that help you relax, reduce pressure, and de-stress, such as spending time in nature, walking, or listening to soft music, you should experience a decrease in heart rate, a reduction in muscular tension, and an improvement in your state of mind.

Boosting Resilience: Continual practice of Christ-centered mindfulness skills (for example, prayer and breath work) can enhance our ability to be more resilient in the face of life's stressors. The more we train our minds to stay present and accept the moment as it is, the more our physiological stress response will be negated.

A Healthier Life: Integrating more mindfulness into our everyday lives has been associated with a whole range of benefits to our mental health, including reducing symptoms of anxiety, depression, or insomnia; improving a general sense of psychological well-being, and increasing our ability to cope with mental health issues.

So, the deal is this: slow down, give thanks, and trust the process. Because when we stop to look up and count our fortunate stars, we find that life is brimming with beauty to enjoy and savor, with treats and tidbits to enjoy along the way, slivers of hope and glimpses of God that can keep hearts beating steadily and grow in whole new directions.

© 2024 - My Peace of Health, LLC

Savoring the little things and making memories that warm the heart.

Aah, it sends such a beautiful message, doesn't it? The quiet goodness of gratitude, of finding peace in the day. The little moments of the day that can be so warming – the ones which happen in between all the in-between getting the bills paid, in between eating something, in between washing something. Just those quiet moments which let us just stop to take a big breath, and connect to ourselves.

Picture yourself in these scenes: sitting at the shore of a still lake, sensing the kiss of rippling water upon your feet, or sitting at home on a comfortable couch in a corner, reclining in the glowing warm light of the candles with a book in one's hands. Moments like these? They're gifts. They calm our minds. They remind us that life can still be good.

Let's just pause, take a deep breath, and savor these moments of peace. They have the power to nourish our spirit, renew our sense of wonder, and remind us to be grateful for the gift of life itself.

And honey, let's not forget trust and submission. God knows what He's doing, so we'd better trust that plan and submit to God's Will in our lives! Things will go wrong, there's no doubt about it. But if instead of fretting and lamenting and wishing upon a star and endlessly rolling those 'whys' around in your mind, choose to pray about it, turn that over fully to God's hands. Say yes to God, then you will be granted that beautiful peaceful feeling that surpasses understanding as it is written: 'Be anxious for nothing, but in everything by prayer and supplication, with thanksgiving, let your requests be made known to God; and the peace of God, which surpasses all understanding, will guard your hearts and minds through Christ Jesus.'

The deal, then, is this: each of us commits to cultivating more gratitude and calmness in our lives, meeting each day with deeply felt gratitude, managing our minds peacefully, counting our blessings, taking time each day in prayer and meditation, and turning to our tribe for support and accountability, cheering each other on.

Building those special family traditions that bring us closer together.

© 2024 - My Peace of Health, LLC

Friday nights in our house? They're practically sacred. As the sun's dipping below the horizon, signaling the start of the weekend and the welcome embrace of the Sabbath—a time for us to unwind, reflect, and truly connect.

We begin with dinner: taco dorados, a family classic that no one ever gets tired of. The smell of corn tortillas sizzling in the pan fills the air, as we gather around the table, setting the stage for an evening of pure joy and gratitude.

As everyone sits down to the meal, we dim the lights, light candles, and put on our worship music. A soft, intimate light fills the room. This little trick helps you enjoy your meal a whole lot more. So do essential oils diffused through our essential oil diffuser. This is the beginning of a sacred, quiet evening.

Eventually, we sit down and dig into our tacos. One by one, we share what has gone well, what has been hard, and the myriad ways in which we've been blessed in the recent week. We laugh together. We listen. We encourage one another across the table through advice and affirmation. Our hearts are all woven closer together.

Following dinner, we circle the piano for the family jam. We might not be Cain the Band or even Maverick City, but our voices come together in a glorious (and not necessarily in perfect tune) cloud of harmony that bathes the space in love and affection. It is a prayer – a song said back to the divine and a means of gathering in unity with each other.

Next comes the devotional – an opportunity to soak up God's goodness and remember the faithfulness of God in the past week. We pop open the Bible, our leaders share some thoughts, we pray and facilitate intercessory petitions, and invite God to respond to and fill our hearts.

Lastly, we stay at home together for a family movie night, all of us on the couch together with popcorn, covered in blankets watching a film that fills our hearts with joy as well as our minds with wisdom.

The credits roll and the night comes to an end. We exchange hugs and kisses, feeling blessed for the time we've spent together that week, and

© 2024 - My Peace of Health, LLC

for all the specialness bestowed upon us by the Sabbath. You see, Friday nights for us weren't a fleeting tradition, a routine – they were a ritual, a communal, loving, spiritual practice; so that while we might be getting closer and closer to each other, heart to heart, week by week, we are also getting closer, once again, to a place beyond us, a place beyond.

And if that doesn't make for a perfect Friday night, I don't know what will. Go get your family and friends together and start building traditions that will last them a lifetime. You won't regret it.

Family therapists and psychologists increasingly stress the role of family rituals and traditions in helping families thrive. Perhaps they'd say something like this:

Family holidays and other rituals allow family members to bond, create shared memories, and engage in family activities. Being part of a ritual can deepen emotional bonds between family members, as well as foster a sense of association (the shared feelings, rituals and memories envelop one in a web of family identity).

A focus on meaningful rituals and routines – for example, family dinners, storytime, book-reading, vacations, and holidays – can offer a sense of stability and predictability, describing familiar patterns that children find comforting and emotionally reassuring. When children know what to expect from a family ritual, they can typically reap the rewards of feeling safe and knowing that their needs are met.

Family rituals and traditions create memorable experiences for family members through special occasions, shared meals, or unique celebrations that family members can reflect on years after the initial event. These shared experiences are something families can reflect upon and engage in such as listening to cherished holiday music, watching favorite movies, or telling stories.

Family rituals offer important communication, reflection, and connection opportunities among family members. For example, sharing stories over dinner, or having a special event such as family game night, offers

© 2024 - My Peace of Health, LLC

opportunities for open communication and connection among family members.

Many family traditions reflect the values, beliefs, and cultural heritage of the family. Parents can use these rituals to instill in their children important values and beliefs they want the child to adopt while helping them develop a cultural identity and a sense of pride in their heritage.

Building these values and beliefs into sustaining family traditions can be a wonderful way to reinforce them in everyday life. Here are some steps you might try:

1. **Reflect on Your Values and Beliefs:** Once you have identified your values and beliefs as a family, take some time to reflect on what they mean to you. Think about what aspects of your culture or religion are the most important to you or where your values intersect with broader questions of meaning and purpose.
2. **Start Small:** Some of the most beautiful traditions are simple, sweet, and small – weekly family dinners, monthly game nights, or yearly camping trips – and they get the job done. Begin with small, doable traditions for your family and work your way up.
3. **Involve Everyone**: Make it a family project to create and maintain your new traditions, ensuring that everyone who wants a say gets one. Encourage open communication and cooperation. Be flexible and considerate in adapting traditions to what is doable for each person at every stage.
4. **Be Consistent:** If you are going to spend the time and energy to create a tradition, make it one that will be revisited and become a fixture in your family life. In other words, they become ritualistic! You especially want your children to recall your family traditions as enduring, so practice them often – whether daily, like the bedtime ritual, or within the same holiday frame, like the Christmas Day activity.
5. **Document Your Memories:** Take pictures, shoot videos, write a journal entry, or put together a scrapbook. You and your loved ones must capture memories of special moments or traditions to create a record of what you hold dear. You might not even realize

© 2024 - My Peace of Health, LLC

how important documenting your memories can be until you see that others don't share your appreciation of such things.

It's more than just making memories and creating traditions; you're creating bonds among your family and infusing your life and your family's life with richness and clarity, for today and for generations to come. Rituals and traditions are precious gifts.

Screen time

Friends, let me have a word with you about technology – that thing, if you will – that's lately been harassing me every waking moment. I, for one, am a huge fan of digital life. I love that we can be instantaneously related more or less across the globe with clicks and keystrokes and swipes and such. But you know what? This relationship, if you will, is all out of whack. The screens are running the show.

I mean – how often do we spend our time constantly checking our phones or tablets, scrolling down social media feeds, or a new series you'd love to watch? We have no time to acknowledge the here-and-now moments – as we are constantly engaged with our phones.

But here's the kicker – when it comes to creating those deep, meaningful connections with our families, sometimes we need to hit the pause button on the screens and tune into each other instead. Trust me, it's worth it.

So what can we do to get the right balance between our love for technology and our love for our kids? The first step is to set some boundaries – a couple of ideas: maybe you choose particular times of the day to have screen-free zones, such as mealtimes or bedtimes – and that includes Mom and Dad too, who are as guilty as anyone!

Second, let's make sure to schedule some screen-free time as a family – a game night, an outdoor excursion, or just sitting in front of a fire sipping hot cocoa and swapping stories. These are the memories we make, the bonds we forge.

© 2024 - My Peace of Health, LLC

And, finally, let's get our imaginative hats on and think of some interesting ways to bring those meaningful connections to life – ways that do not rely on having multiple devices turned on at once. How about instituting a family book club – working our way through a new story together every week to read before bed every night? Or how about a weekly arts-and-crafts night – where we get to practice some creativity and come up with interesting things to work on together? The world is our oyster!

In the end, therefore, it's all about mixing in a healthy dose of technology with a good dose of human, face-to-face contact with your loved ones. Away from the screens, and people, and once again I say: let's go make some memories.

Child development specialists are likely to emphasize the value of controlling screen time for children's well-being. Here's how they might explain it:

Research Perspective: Spending too much time using screen devices, often associated with the digital age, is having important consequences for children's development. Too much screen time, especially in younger children, can interfere with their social and emotional development and cognition, as well as their physical health. This includes the development of face-to-face social interactions, empathy, and emotional self-control.

Making Boundaries: Help kids stay within safe guidelines for screen time appropriate to their age. Give specific limits on time spent watching entertainment content versus educational content. Make family zones, like dining areas and bedrooms, 'zero screens' zones.

Encouraging Diverse Activities: Encouraging children to play outdoors, read, draw, paint, cook, do, help, etc., is important for their psychological and physical health. Outdoor play, family gatherings, practicing creative and artistic hobbies, reading, board games, sports, and other leisure activities might give children more opportunities to communicate, cooperate, and have fun than just sitting in front of screens.

Lead by example: urge parents and other caregivers to be model screen citizens. They can practice mindful screen-life habits and establish limits,

© 2024 - My Peace of Health, LLC

and they can also restrict their own screen time and pay attention to other people while they're around.

Promoting Open Dialogue: Make a dialogue with the children about the world regarding screen time. Explain the rationale behind limiting screen time, teach them the dangers of misusing it, and involve them in the decision-making process about setting rules regarding screen-based activities. This equips them with important decision-making skills to use independently.

In other words, good screen time practice includes setting limits, encouraging other activities, modeling the behavior you want to see, and keeping communication open. By setting priorities with screen habits and also for time outside of the digital world, we can help children develop into their best digital selves.

Let's make a conscious effort to create enduring memories for your family and each of your loved ones, memorable, bittersweet, loving, fleeting, or meaningful experiences that bond you intimately for years to come. The screens can wait. Turn them off. Get the kids involved, now and again. Now, go out and play.

The connection between mind and body

The integration of the mind and body forms a crucial concept of holistic wellness, one that understands that our mental, emotional, and physical states are interdependent: how we think and feel impacts our physical health, and likewise, how we feel physically impacts our mental and emotional state.

When we feel under stress or anxious or have other negative emotions, our bodies often react with physical symptoms, such as muscle tension, headaches, or gastrointestinal issues. On the flip side, chronic physical ills or imbalances can lead us to feel frustrated, sad, or anxious.

Paying attention to what our bodies tell us – how they feel and in which ways they react – can help us attend to our own needs. Hearing our aching joints or tight stomachs, and noticing our tears or lack of energy, can assist us in making appropriate self-care choices.

© 2024 - My Peace of Health, LLC

1. Prioritizing self-care practices that nourish both mind and body is essential for women seeking to maintain balance and promote overall well-being. Here's how these practices align with Christian values:

2. Eating Well: focusing on nourishing food stems from the Christian stewardship of the body (1 Corinthians 6:19-20), understood as a temple of the Holy Spirit. A balanced diet based on fruits, vegetables, whole grains, and plant proteins allows you to value God's gift of health and life.

3. Stress Management: Stress-reduction techniques practice the Christian value of trusting in God's provision and finding rest in Him (Matthew 11:28-30). Deep breathing, meditation practice, and prayer are techniques you can use to let go of the tensions in your body and allow yourself to rest in God and His sovereignty.

4. Higher Quality Sleep: Because sleep is a lifestyle issue dealing with the Sabbath rest and restoration which God intended for us (Genesis 2:2-3), a good way to create higher quality sleep is to build a spiritual 'sleep hygiene' practice into bedtime. Reading Scripture, praying and talking to God about the events of the day, and pausing to put things into a God-centered perspective, can drastically change the quality of sleep.

5. Healthy expression: Managing emotions in healthy ways aligns with the biblical call to cast our burdens on the Lord; for He cares for us (Psalm 55:22, 1 Peter 5:7). Journaling, art therapy, or talking with a trusted counselor or fellow sister in Christ can all be beneficial ways for Christian women to healthily express their emotions through their faith.

These holistic self-care practices can bring you closer to God and enable you to embrace your inner life's depth and connectedness if integrated into your life daily. With these dual paths to living, you can lead life more fully, honestly, and intentionally, integrating the knowledge and spirit of your faith into your wellness.

© 2024 - My Peace of Health, LLC

Discussion Questions

1. When were you last in a place of quiet? What happened then? How did it make you feel?

2. Think of a time when the noise and clatter of life became too much. How did you deal with your reaction? What could you do next time to cope?

© 2024 - My Peace of Health, LLC

3. What are some family traditions and rituals that warm your heart and bring you closer to your loved ones? Are there any that you would like to start?

4. Reflect on your family's overall relationship with technology and screen time. How does it function between family members, and how does it exclude people? How much time is spent on screens at home? In what ways could you reclaim more of the time you're seeking from technology?

© 2024 - My Peace of Health, LLC

© 2024 - My Peace of Health, LLC

© 2024 - My Peace of Health, LLC

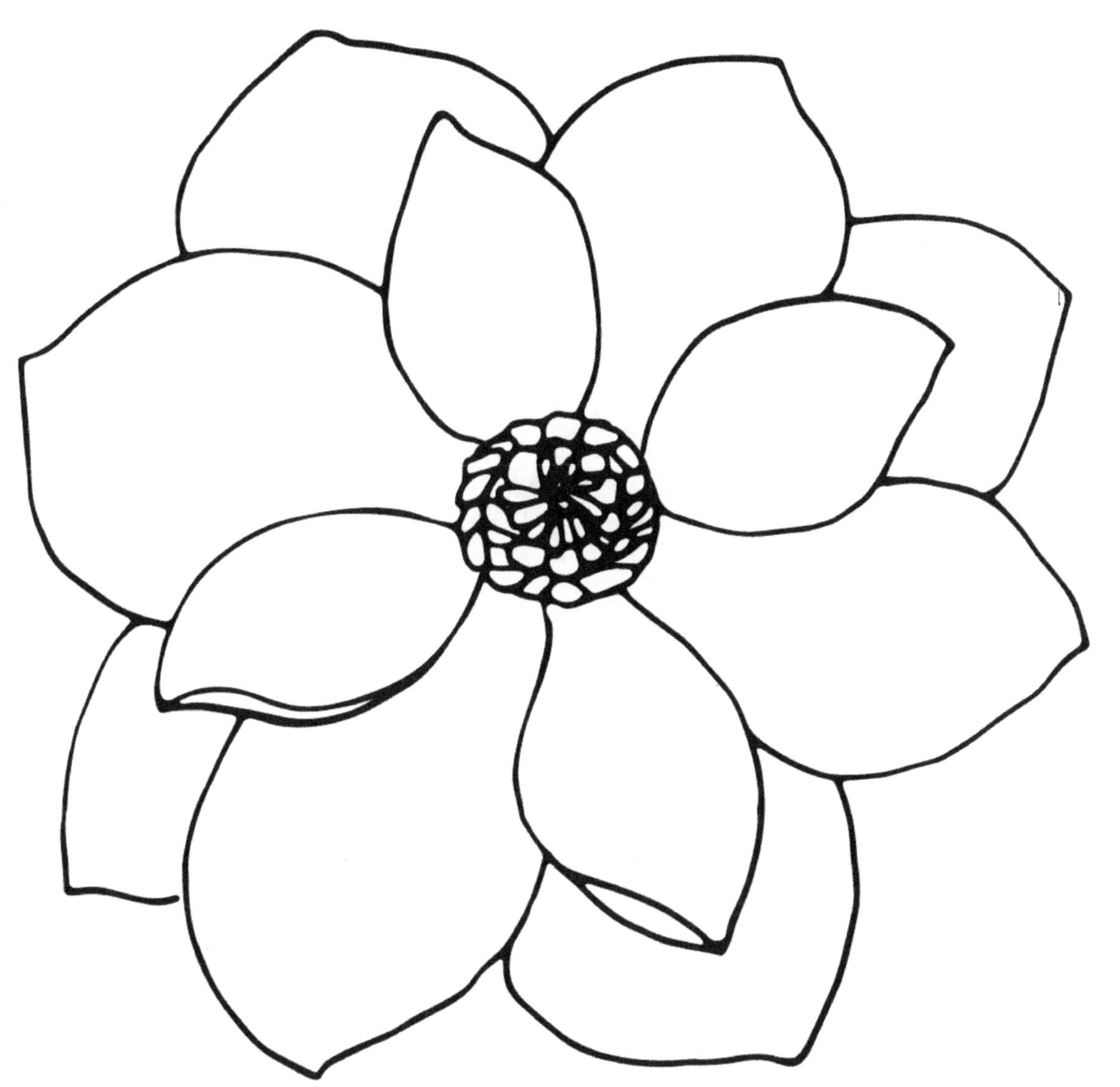

© 2024 - My Peace of Health, LLC

Chapter 8

Testimony of Faith

My favorite story, told many times by my father, illustrates my grandmother as a symbol of toughness and resilience. She was a pregnant widow with a two-year-old, then remarried, had four boys, and escaped domestic violence. However, she refused to be defined by that pain.

At 35, with six children, she defied the odds and determined that there was nothing in her path that she couldn't alter. She went back to school to become a nurse. Some said that she couldn't. But she could.

He'd tell stories about the struggles she faced, how she worked hard, and how she never stopped believing in God. Her story became an example for the family, a reminder that nothing is impossible with God.

My grandmother's affirmation taught me the value of resilience, to never give up on one's dream. Her strength and tenacity in the face of adversity have inspired me to this day to press on. And even though it was difficult to change, I continue to tell myself that with God, all things are possible.

As I think about her life, I'm reminded of the many stories of faith that both surround and sustain me as I do all that I do. Every testimony, at the altar or around the dinner table, is an act of faith. It declares God's love and the transforming power of human perseverance.

Therefore, when I give you my story, recognizing that it is not just mine but woven from the testimonies of so many others, before me and after me, and with this, may you learn to believe that, with God, nothing is impossible; we are never alone; He walks with us; He feeds us; He sustains us; He carries us; He prepares for us a place of rest and wages eternal with Him, where we will be whole, and one day we will walk with Him in the glory of Heaven!

© 2024 - My Peace of Health, LLC

My Testimony

My family was the foundation of my faith from the beginning. My mother was a health educator and devoted Christian who taught me reverence for the house of our Lord and the love of his people just like her mother and grandmother; she taught me to lift my face to him in song, in summer and winter alike. When life got dark, I watched as she clung to her love for God so that when life twisted us in knots, her faith could act like a magnet pulling back the invasion of bitterness. Trials could come, but she wouldn't waver; she was stronger than her challenges, and because of that, she was stronger than those challenges for me too.

And I learned other lessons from my father also— a soldier turned art teacher and like his mother, a prayer warrior, whose life is an example of how learning and prayer can both help you, while also finding a way to articulate his love of God in his artwork and poetry.

In the quiet moments, I recall my mother's silent tears as she pulled the car to the side of the road, the strains of "The Battle is the Lord's" echoing through the radio. Though she never vocalized her pain, her silent communion with the Healer spoke volumes.

I especially recall silently observing my father as he was bent over his desk, he read and prayed, clinging to his craft as a way of his expression of faith.

I began to learn again, through their steadfast faith, about the reliability of God's character. I discovered that I could take heart from their unspoken testimonies: that God restores, that God heals, that God alone makes our suffering worthwhile, and that He hadn't changed in the millennia since their creation. In their lives I found comfort, and in their steadfast faith, I discovered courage for my own.

But, still there I sat, the waterworks in full swing. 19 years old and utterly helpless. My 3-year-old son looked at me from the back seat. 'Mommy,' he asked. 'Why are you crying?' Somewhere among the jumble of

© 2024 - My Peace of Health, LLC

parental instincts, my heart was blinking to remind me: be strong for his sake. 'Jesus gonna heal it,' he had said. He just knew.

For the first time in my life, I felt a huge sense of parental responsibility. My 'assignment' was to myself and my children. I was to be their missionary, teaching them, building their faith, and leading them into truth. 'Mommy' was not my identity, it was an appointment, a privilege, and an honor. It was a gift from God.

Yet as my son's words rang out, I shrank inside with the faint echo of my shortcomings. I am not like them. Not like my mother and father, not like a long line of grandmothers and other women I held in high esteem whose steadfast faith seemed to me a superpower, a strength that I could never reach. I felt fragile and like an inadequate parent.

I wept and wept. I unburdened everything to my Creator, my Carrier of tears, the only One who could understand. It was my steering wheel, my altar, my sacred space, I was in the presence of the greatest intimacy with God, where I poured out my fears, all of my insecurities, and my self-doubt before Him. It was the knowledge of God's great strength in my weakness, made perfect.

Years later, after that divine appointment, God, hearing my prayers, sent me a travel partner for this life, my husband Simon, whom I have relied on for being the refuge in the middle of any storm and for enabling my faith in God and myself to grow and not give up in the face of the toughest nights. We built a family and home together – a gift of God and love that does not allow even the darkest of nights to prevail.

Nevertheless, the road has not been without its challenges. Our last few years were admittedly horrible, and two years ago topped the cake when my eldest daughter nearly took her life.

I distinctly recall how, 17 years earlier, when she was only six weeks old, I sat in the car sobbing as she was there next to her brother, and now, as I looked at her, a sweet teen struggling with her grief, I mentally saw the image of a reflection of my younger self. History repeating itself, I stood there in the reality of her hurt. Once again, I found myself burdened by

© 2024 - My Peace of Health, LLC

mom guilt, questioning my ability to fill my role, as I mentally went down the list of ways that I felt I had failed.

Leaving her side momentarily, I found myself consumed by the letter she had written, its words etched into my mind like a dagger. I longed for peace, the same hope that sustained my cousin Wilma Rudolph, the strength of my great-grandmother, the resilience of my grandmothers, and the peace that enveloped my parents. Yet, in the discord of doubt and despair, all I could muster was a single word: "Jesus."

As tears streamed down my face, I cried out to the Peace Speaker, seeking solace in His comforting embrace. And in that moment of brokenness, my three-year-old daughter echoed her brother's words, "Mommy, why are you crying? Jesus will heal her because that is what Jesus does." Her tiny voice was a beacon of unwavering faith during our storm.

That night, my understanding of love was incalculable, just like the Father's love for us in sending His Son. The storm will still rage on, and I know I will still feel the beating waves of it, but now I know that the Commander of the winds and the waves, is with me, beside me, and I rest my weary heart.

So, my friend, as I share my journey with you, I want you to know that finding peace is not just a possibility—it's a promise. My Peace of Health was created because of a deep desire to help women and families like yours discover that peace is within reach.

Whatever the storms around you, whatever state you might be in, Christ is knocking at the door of your heart. He desires to come in and gently heal all brokenness you experience, in all dimensions of your existence. Is it not beautiful? My dear, let us walk as one towards this place of peace. We are not alone.

Here are some practical tips for nurturing faith and resilience in daily life:

1. **Daily Prayer and Meditation**: Set aside some time to pray and/or meditate each day. Let your prayer be a quiet moment, an expression of thanks, a plea for guidance, a communion with

© 2024 - My Peace of Health, LLC

God. Regular prayer and meditation can create a lasting relationship with God within your heart. They can bring you inner strength and peace.

2. **Scripture Reading and Reflection:** Cultivate a regular practice of reading and reflecting on scripture. Select verses that relate to where you are in life or what you're seeking God for and think about how that particular verse applies to your situation. Meditate on it. What do these verses mean for me?

3. **Journal**: Keep a journal to write out your prayers and reflections. Writing, as a spiritual discipline, is beneficial for processing your emotions, expressing gratitude, and monitoring your spiritual development. Make sure to also use your journal as a self-checking mechanism to write out your answered prayers and moments of spiritual growth.

4. **Ask for Help:** When you have questions or doubts, talk to mentors, spiritual leaders, or counselors. Ask them for prayer and support. If life is difficult, ask a friend or family member to pray for you or to listen to you. You don't have to struggle alone.

5. **Gratitude Practice:** Practice gratitude by intentionally focusing on what you are thankful for in your life. At the beginning of every day, express gratitude for the gift of life and your health, for loving and supportive relationships, and for the things and people that you love. Keep a gratitude journal or learn some gratitude prayers to nurture a positive outlook and attitude.

As I reflect on the faith walk of deliverance and redemption chronicled in this chapter, I am compelled to pause and give thanks to the systems of support that facilitated my existence through the darkest of seasons in my life. The Bible teaches us to give thanks, and I want to pause and thank every individual who has been instrumental in my journey.

I would like to extend appreciation to all the officers and paramedics who responded, and to the nurses, doctors and therapist who cared for my daughter in the ambulance and Emergency Room. Without your expertise, professionalism, and kindness, I fear our daughter would not be alive today.

© 2024 - My Peace of Health, LLC

To my friends on whom I can count: Thank you for your boundless affection, your prayers, hugs, and caring support, for listening, crying with me, and encouraging me — always you have been there when I called. I would not be here without any one of you.

Acknowledging my gratitude to those of you in Stand Unshaken, Soul Sisters, and Melanated Mamas, I express appreciation for the support networks that people created to promote well-being, self-care, and companionship among people facing adversity and uncertainty.

Dr. Karla Montague-Brown, your wisdom, guidance, and words of comfort have been a beacon of light on my journey. Thank you for your time, your books, and your empowering words that have helped me navigate through the storm.

To my beloved brother and sister, Mom and Dad, your unwavering support, strength, and unconditional love have been a constant source of encouragement and reassurance. I am blessed to have you by my side, cheering me on every step of the way.

And to my wonderful children, you are the delight of my life and my greatest teacher. Thank you for loving me and keeping me sane through all of life's madness.

Simon, my husband, your love, support, and sacrifice have taken us through not just this moment but many, through the darkest night and tearful cries. Thank you for always being there for us, for me, for our family, our children, even when your strength was down.

Furthermore, a special word of thanks to the many platforms and ministries that have allowed me to share my testimony over the past year – it is your readiness to give a voice to what I'm sharing with you here that has enabled the gospel of hope and faith to be transmitted to so many more.

Finally, I offer my deepest gratitude to the Lord, who has been my Peace and my Rock throughout it all. Thank you for granting me peace of mind, body, and soul, and for allowing me to rest in Your unfailing love.

© 2024 - My Peace of Health, LLC

It is with this feeling of gratitude that I think back to the Gospel story of Jesus curing the lepers. After being healed, only one came back to thank Jesus. Similarly, like the thankful leper, I want to go back and say, 'Thanks.' Thanks to all of you who have touched my life with your goodness, love, and support.

Thanks to you all and God bless you.

A Prayer For You

And now, this moment of prayer comes to a close, but may we take the sense of communion and petition into all future moments.

Heavenly Father,

In life's storms and trials, we come before You with open hearts and bowed spirits.

Thank you for Your unwavering love and grace that carry us through challenges.

I lift those who are hurting, broken, and alone. Bring healing to their hearts, and peace to their minds.

Grant us the courage to surrender fears to you, the ultimate healer. Help us trust your timing and promises, even in uncertainty.

Guide us as we journey through life's twists, leading us into truth and light. May we spread Your love and peace in a thirsty world.

Grant us wisdom and discernment, that we may honor Your name. Help us to live peaceful and purposeful lives in Your Spirit.

We praise you, Lord, for You alone are worthy of honor and glory. Help our lives reflect Your goodness and grace.

In Jesus' name,

Amen.

© 2024 - My Peace of Health, LLC

Here are some additional scriptural references that align with the themes of faith, resilience, and gratitude:

- **Philippians 4:6-7:** Do not be anxious about anything, but in every situation, by prayer and petition, with thanksgiving, present your requests to God. And the peace of God, which transcends all understanding, will guard your hearts and your minds in Christ Jesus.
- **Psalm 23:4:** Even though I walk through the darkest valley, I will fear no evil, for you are with me; your rod and your staff, they comfort me.
- **Romans 8:28:** And we know that in all things God works for the good of those who love him, who have been called according to his purpose.
- **2 Corinthians 12:9-10:** But he said to me, 'My grace is sufficient for you, for my power is made perfect in weakness.' Therefore I will boast all the more gladly about my weaknesses, so that Christ's power may rest on me. That is why, for Christ's sake, I delight in weaknesses, in insults, in hardships, in persecutions, in difficulties. For when I am weak, then I am strong.
- **Hebrews 10:24-25:** And let us consider how we may spur one another on toward love and good deeds, not giving up meeting together, as some are in the habit of doing, but encouraging one another—and all the more as you see the Day approaching.

© 2024 - My Peace of Health, LLC

Discussion Questions:

1. Share a time when you experienced God's faithfulness in your life.

2. How can we encourage each other, especially when we are struggling?

© 2024 - My Peace of Health, LLC

3. Think of how crucial it is to open our hands: to release that fear and that struggle, and to place them in God's hands, trusting that he will put every broken thing back in its rightful place.

Disclaimer: Suicide Prevention

Please, if you or someone you know is struggling, get help now. In the US, call the National Suicide Prevention Lifeline at 1-800-273-TALK (1-800-273-8255) for free and confidential support 24 hours a day, seven days a week. Just remember, people love and care about you. Don't be afraid to reach out and ask for support.

© 2024 - My Peace of Health, LLC

© 2024 - My Peace of Health, LLC

© 2024 - My Peace of Health, LLC

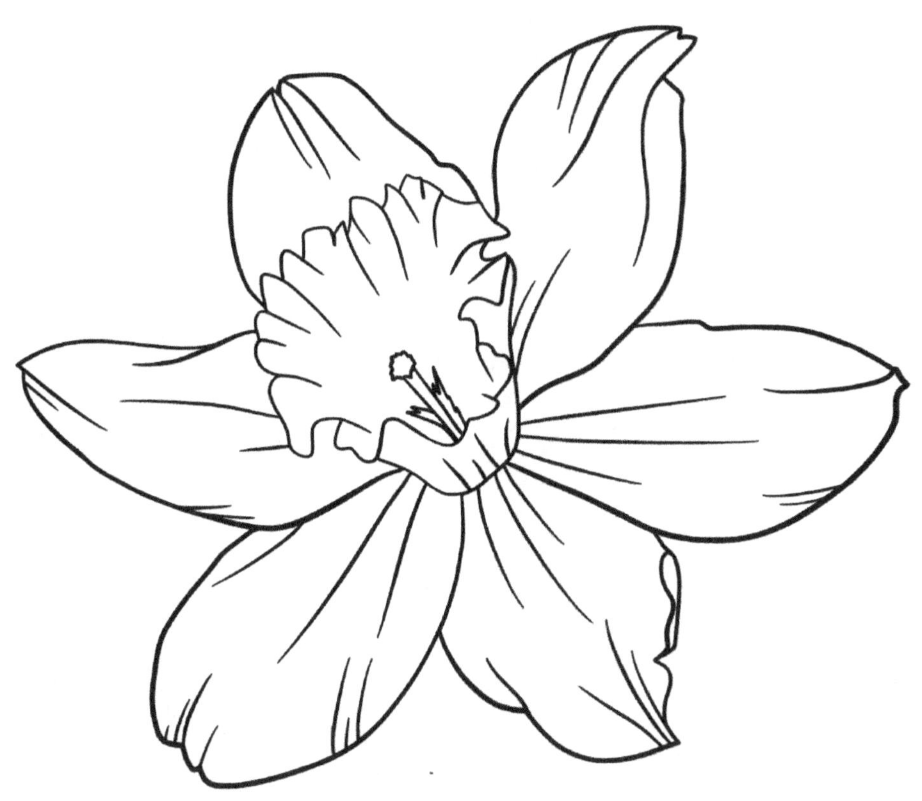

© 2024 - My Peace of Health, LLC

© 2024 - My Peace of Health, LLC

Chapter 9

Embracing Change

Approaching change is about the greatest adventure you can ever have, right? Of course, it is! Life growth, evolution, finding the treasures hidden in that scary place just beyond the limits of your comfort zone. But this is where we live folks, which means that, not surprisingly, hanging in mid-air with no safety net whilst being propelled on a crazy ride into the great unknown can also be a wild ride into the great unknown.

But I said the change process can be hard. However, that uncertainty – that openness, if you prefer – brings with it a great opportunity to settle into a trusted environment for release, growth, and change… as both you and your situation evolve. Cutting ties with the usual – whether from a job, an apartment, or a city – means new experiences, new suggestions, and new options. It's about moving past what you know and into a quickly backfilled ocean of unfilled space, trusting that God is helping you down the stairs.

Think of every shift, every season of regeneration, as a white piece of paper waiting for you to make your mark. A chance to depart from would-be losses and to paint your life; to let go of what no longer serves you and rise to your magnificent self – your next portrait of yourself.

Let's start with the messy truth of change – it is not always sunshine and rainbows. Sometimes it is truly messy and uncomfortable and just downright challenging. But it's in those sticky, messy moments of change that we grow the most. We find our grit and our resilience as we embrace the uncomfortable, lean into the uncertainty, and push through fear.

It reminded me of when change came to my life, unasked: when that momentous feeling that something is about to happen or has already happened infiltrated my consciousness; that moment when I can feel, but cannot see, a major change is on the horizon; a tumultuous time when my life was in shambles, when nothing was certain, and when the balance teetered like crumbly dunes.

© 2024 - My Peace of Health, LLC

Everything in my life had been based on the assumption that everything was going to stay the same. And guilty as charged: I had rationalized a mundane existence based on continuity and repetition. My fear of change was real.

At first, I resisted changing, sticking to what was familiar. Why just go back to normal? But for me to live – not just to exist – I had to learn to embrace change.

But as I became willing to take risks and push beyond my comfort zone, not only has energy entered my life but also real purpose. Trying new moves at the gym, experimenting in the kitchen with a new plant-based dish, starting new friendships, or welcoming new clients professionally, has brought energy and renewal.

Only, I have to admit, it wasn't always easy when the future was a big black hole frightening me when self-doubt crept up on me, and when I wondered if I had what it took to navigate through the treacherous currents of change.

And yet, it was in mind-bending moments that I experienced some of the richest lessons in personal transformation. We become our most powerful when we move through the discomfort, go beyond our fears, and choose to tolerate the uncertainty.

What began as something to be tolerated had transformed into something new to be welcomed, into something that could bring about fulfillment and a rich life.

In the process of embracing the new, I learned that it's acceptable to be afraid, to fall, and to make mistakes. But, most importantly, it's important to be brave and keep moving – one step at a time – knowing that there is always something beautiful that will blossom from each change.

Joyce came to me plagued by an abiding terror of change. She was engaged to her college boyfriend, whom she thought she could spend her life with, and her fears of change and loss were so enormous that she was spending her days trying to vanquish them with a slew of

© 2024 - My Peace of Health, LLC

temporary fixes. Late nights and rapid weight-loss diets proved to be as frustrating and irritating as the fear they were trying to overcome.

In coaching sessions, I asked Joyce to imaginatively go deeper into her goals and discover what she truly wanted for good health and a good life. While the prospect of failure was terrifying, the prospect of success stopped her cold in her tracks. It meant a new life. A healthy life. A life of joy and family and activity.

As a team, we continued taking small, easy-to-handle steps toward healthful change, making it happen a little at a time. Plant foods, restful sleep, meditative spiritual readings, outdoor walks with fresh air and sunlight – Joyce moved from one change to the next, and the transformation began to take hold. I help people embrace a healthy lifestyle by choosing healthful food, daily activity, water, sunshine, sober living, fresh air, rest, and faith.

Joyce's confidence grew in tandem with her ability to face her fears. On the morning of her dress shopping, she was terrified. When she stepped on the scale, she had lost 15 lbs in eight weeks and was close to goal. With each weigh-in, Joyce started to recognize change as something she no longer needed to fear but as an opportunity to transform, to become filled, and to live again.

Whenever you feel the breeze of your inner metamorphosis, you are not alone, God is with you, encouraging you, guiding you, hugging and encouraging you in that process of change.

And in all the kicking and screaming about what is changing, and all the turning around to have a last glimpse of what is passing away, stop. Simply stop. Breathe. Lean into the moment. Hear the quiet in the storm. Listen for God, speaking His still, small voice in your heart. There, you will discover the grace and beauty of this remarkable life.

Here's some expert advice on the topic of embracing change:

Dr. Carol Dweck (Psychologist, Stanford University):

© 2024 - My Peace of Health, LLC

One of the world's experts in this area is the psychologist Dr. Carol Dweck at Stanford University, who has researched mindset extensively and coined the terms 'fixed' and 'growth' mindsets. Dweck claims that we are all either in a fixed mindset or a growth mindset. 'People in a fixed mindset believe their basic abilities, their intelligence, their talents, are just fixed traits,' she explains. 'They have a certain amount, and that's that, and then their goal becomes to look smart all the time and also to – God forbid – look dumb sometimes, or on occasion not know something. They don't want to expose their lack of knowledge. They're afraid that will reveal that they're not as smart as other people and that people will think less of them. Whereas people with a growth mindset believe their basic traits, such as their intelligence or their talents, can develop with effort, practice, and good teaching. Because of that, they allow themselves to be vulnerable in a way.

Brene Brown (Researcher, Author, Speaker):

The work of Brene Brown, the social worker and researcher of courage, vulnerability, and wholehearted living, can be a helpful guide to developing courage and presence amid change: Move toward your vulnerabilities. Let go of who you think you should be and dare to live and lead from your whole heart. Choosing courage over comfort is never easy. Waking up to a reality that might be different than your expectations is tough. However, in the pain of the vulnerable moment – embracing uncertainty, loneliness, scarcity, and imperfection – lies the seed of transformation and renewal. Embracing vulnerability and the resulting courage brings new creative landscapes and a unique brand of authenticity and will to life.

Dr. Dan Siegel (Psychiatrist, Author):

Using Dan Siegel's interpersonal neurobiology approach as a model, we can start to see the value of integrative flexibility of mind to handle change. This involves a process that he calls 'mindsight', enabling one to develop an increasingly clear and tangible 'window' on internal experiences, so that we can bring to mind insights and greater clarity to our often fraught inner life. Now we are moving beyond being aware and present to ourselves and into the realm of action goals and trajectories.

© 2024 - My Peace of Health, LLC

Bringing that steadiness of center to our lives supports us through big changes and helps us to build that all-important attribute of resilience.

So, on an optimistic note, here are some empowering steps you can take to turn change into significant opportunities for peaceful growth and transformation:

1. **Change is Inevitable**: Let's view it not as a burden but as a blessing. Let's permit ourselves to say goodbye to the past with tenderness while intentionally creating anew.
2. **Be Rooted:** Be rooted in our relationship with God, in those values by which we aspire to live with integrity; and be rooted in something even more solid than these, namely in what we surely are, in the truth of who we are. Choose practices that ground you, whether it be in prayer, studying Scripture, or nature.
3. **Self-Compassion**: Moving through change can be challenging. But remember, we are humans and need to be forgiving towards ourselves. Allow for grace. You don't have to change the way you are feeling but know that whatever you feel during change is OK. You may respond in all or some of the ways suggested, and that also is OK. How did you fare?
4. **Circle Up:** Gather your tribe of encouraging sisters; lean into your family, friends, coaches, or mentors to be your walking partners, cheerleaders, and wise sages.
5. **Open Up Your Mind:** We might not like change but that doesn't mean we won't embrace it with curiosity and readiness to learn and grow. A world of opportunity for personal and professional development awaits, just around the corner of our comfort zone. Be brave enough to try anything once.
6. **Set your intentions:** Hold in your heart or articulate in your mind your biggest hopes for what you want to create or reinvent through this process. Be clear about your goals – what you desire to experience, accomplish, and become – and follow them with dedicated and inspired action.
7. **FLEXIBILITY IS PARAMOUNT:** My dearest, remember, flexibility is our best friend, so we will embrace it, especially when it comes to changes in our plans. We will adjust, knowing that we are

© 2024 - My Peace of Health, LLC

being guided by the Lord and that He will take us down a much better road.

8. **Cultivate Gratitude:** As we approach inquisitiveness, let's nurture a grateful, grateful heart for what change has brought to you – chances and lessons – even as its winds continue blowing and you navigate often unexpected twists and turns on the bent-over path of an oak.

9. **Connect With Your Source:** As this journey takes place, take with you an indestructible line to your Source – to faith and the loving presence of God. Lean upon Him for strength, be directed by Him, and take comfort in Him, for He is with you, holding you close every step of the way.

10. **Celebrate the small victories:** Life is full of small steps in the right direction. Be enthusiastic and celebrate small victories.

And remember sister, that you're stronger than you think, that by standing amid change with faith and patience, your 'expectancy will be filled with overflowing forever and ever.'

It's time to grab the reins and welcome change as a chance for a peaceful evolution and transformation. Don't wait for a better moment, or for all the stars to be aligned – do it now, wherever you are. Stop and ponder interior changes going on in your life, and how they can proceed even more smoothly and peacefully. The changes will happen, but how you deal with them is quite up to you.

Commit to showing yourself kindness, seeking support from your community, and staying rooted in your faith as you navigate through change. Set meaningful goals, stay adaptable, and foster an attitude of gratitude for the journey ahead.

In the end, trust God to figure out your journey and hold onto his hope for you. Trust him to provide the power and the direction, to lead you through whatever it takes to cultivate the most compassionate, attractive, and fruitful life you can. And then trust him to do the work that will bring you through this uncertainty and change with freshness, with fortitude, and with forceful flourishing.

© 2024 - My Peace of Health, LLC

Thus, are you ready to walk courageously into the unknown and embrace the parameters of change with peace and grace? The journey ahead awaits – let us walk together there, in faith and peace.

Strengthening our bonds and facing challenges together.

Her name was Ruth. Here was a poor Moabite widow who had married one of Naomi's sons. Naomi's husband and both of her sons had died, making her a widow with two daughters-in-law, Orpah and Ruth. Naomi was moving back to her husband's people in Bethlehem. She told her daughters-in-law to return to their people.

Orpah went home to her family while Ruth stayed on and committed herself, in some of the best-known words of Bible loyalty, to Naomi: 'Where you go I will go, and where you stay I will stay. Your people will be my people and your God my God' (Ruth 1:16).

Obligated to Naomi, this Moabitess turned to Bethlehem and came to live in the country that was scattered across the face of Palaestina. She was a foreigner in the land. In foreign territory, Ruth took Naomi as herself and labored to support them both. Through her hard labor, she gleaned in the field of Boaz, a rich landowner, and eventually caught his affections for him.

Boaz was so pleased with Ruth's virtue and her loyalty to Naomi that he was generous to her. He redeemed Naomi's piece of property by marrying Ruth and, with Obed, their son, they became ancestors of King David and therefore, ultimately, of Jesus Christ.

The story of Ruth and Naomi reveals how resiliency, flexibility, and unity can overcome practically insurmountable obstacles. In losing her husband and leaving her home behind for a foreign culture, Ruth remained steadfast in her support of Naomi. As a result of their unity, Ruth found financial security and marital happiness beyond her wildest dreams.

We learn from this couple that we can support the ones we love, even at the greatest risk, and that we can expect a future from God that is better than we can imagine. Through life's unexpected curves and bends, a

© 2024 - My Peace of Health, LLC

family's resilience or adaptability is strained. They may do so but emerge more closely bound than ever before.

Resilience is the capacity to bounce back. This quality should be nurtured in all members of the family. Encourage members to talk about their feelings and problems, to practice empathy, and to find solutions to problems together. Let them know that they can't always avoid storms, but they can be ready for these challenging moments. This enables the family to provide mutual support in dealing with storms.

Flexibility is another important factor for family harmony, especially with the unceasing evolution of our society. Don't be afraid to be flexible and open to new ideas, cultures, and ways of thinking. Encourage your family members to embrace change as a positive experience to expand their world, not as a threat but as an opportunity to develop and progress. As family members adapt to new situations together, they demonstrate the strength of the family as one cohesive unit.

Unity is what holds a family together and is the source of togetherness, security, and love. In your family, promote a culture of unity. Spend quality time together: go on fun outings as a group, have conversations at the dinner table, and do things together. Make sure that you are all there to support and nurture each other. Celebrate each other's achievements and celebrate as a family. Encourage everyone to work together collaboratively – 'we are greater together than we are apart'.

When adversity strikes, a family's resilience, flexibility, and togetherness shine most brightly. By cultivating resilience, flexibility, and connection within your family, you will create a sturdy foundation for your family to weather the storms in life while coming out on the other side stronger, closer, and more resilient than ever. So, do your part. Start here: strengthening these cornerstones of family life.

© 2024 - My Peace of Health, LLC

Here are some verses to meditate on or highlight in your free time.

Isaiah 43:18-19: "Forget the former things; do not dwell on the past. See, I am doing a new thing! Now it springs up; do you not perceive it? I am making a way in the wilderness and streams in the wasteland."

Jeremiah 29:1: "For I know the plans I have for you," declares the Lord, "plans to prosper you and not to harm you, plans to give you hope and a future."

Psalm 27:1: "The Lord is my light and my salvation— whom shall I fear? The Lord is the stronghold of my life— of whom shall I be afraid?"

Proverbs 3:5-6: "Trust in the Lord with all your heart and lean not on your understanding; in all your ways submit to him, and he will make your paths straight."

2 Corinthians 5:17: "Therefore, if anyone is in Christ, the new creation has come: The old has gone, the new is here!"

Ecclesiastes 3:1: "There is a time for everything and a season for every activity under the heavens."

Philippians 4:6-7: "Do not be anxious about anything, but in every situation, by prayer and petition, with thanksgiving, present your requests to God. And the peace of God, which transcends all understanding, will guard your hearts and your minds in Christ Jesus."

Romans 8:28: "And we know that in all things God works for the good of those who love him, who have been called according to his purpose."

Hebrews 13:8: "Jesus Christ is the same yesterday and today and forever."

Joshua 1:9: "Have I not commanded you? Be strong and courageous. Do not be afraid; do not be discouraged, for the Lord your God will be with you wherever you go."

© 2024 - My Peace of Health, LLC

Coaching Questions:

Resilience:

1. When challenges arise, how do you usually respond? What helps you bounce back?

2. Think back to the tough times you've faced. How did those experiences shape your resilience?

© 2024 - My Peace of Health, LLC

3. Who might you reach out to when you need a little help? How might you grow your web of support?

4. When you encounter a setback or experience a key life event, how do you interpret these things as learning experiences for growing into a better or fuller version of yourself?

© 2024 - My Peace of Health, LLC

Adaptability:

1. Are you a shifter or a settler? Are you comfortable with change, or do you prefer stability? Which strategies do you have for adjusting to new situations?

2. Reflect on a significant change you've successfully navigated. What lessons did you learn?

3. In your daily life, how can you cultivate a more flexible mindset?

© 2024 - My Peace of Health, LLC

Unity:

1. What steps do you take to foster unity in your relationships?

2. How does effective communication contribute to unity within your family or group?

© 2024 - My Peace of Health, LLC

3. Are there any conflicts or challenges hindering unity? How can you address them constructively?

4. How do you celebrate and embrace diversity in your community or organization?

These questions help you to identify where you are heading in terms of positive growth and change as a result of how you respond to adversity, how well you've adapted to your circumstances, and how deeply you value your relationships.

© 2024 - My Peace of Health, LLC

© 2024 - My Peace of Health, LLC

© 2024 - My Peace of Health, LLC

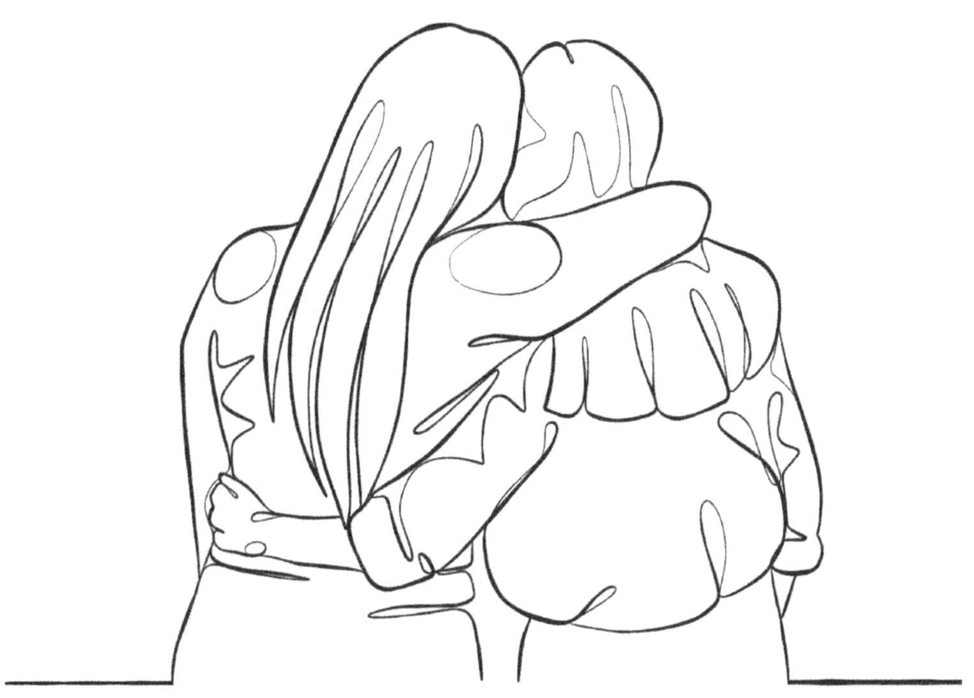

© 2024 - My Peace of Health, LLC

© 2024 - My Peace of Health, LLC

And with that, my darling, we draw to an end of this incredible journey that I have been so privileged to embark on with all of you, dear readers. We have delved into the frailties of womanhood and examined the workings of our families, and our collective ability to navigate the joy of living in harmony with ourselves and with one another. To each and everyone – a big thank you!

And let's permit ourselves to celebrate the wins, ride out the waves, and honor the strength and resilience that lives in all of us. We've come together with a unified and noble effort to live lives that are whole, joyful and sane, and as we put this book to rest, my heart is full of hope and thanks for the astonishing peace we've found.

May I simply say that as long as you keep walking in the light of His peace and grace of the Spirit, you'll never be disconnected from the beauty and the power that is splattered all over you? You are wonderfully and marvelously made and you'll never lose the uniqueness of your personality and talent, your ingenuity and strength, your beauty and voice – your awesome difference.

Let your days be blessed. Let them be filled with love, gladness, and an unfathomable peace that no one can take away from you. You are not alone. The One who created you loves you with everlasting love.

Thanks from the bottom of my heart for letting me be a part of it. And cheers to living every moment full-out, with the fullness of your heart and love, and radiating peace and happiness as you go.

And please, if you are feeling up for keeping the journey moving, visit me over at My Peace of Health coaching services. We work with women, and their families, like you every day – women who want true peace of mind in every aspect of life.

With love and endless gratitude,

Candice Leanos

© 2024 - My Peace of Health, LLC

© 2024 - My Peace of Health, LLC

Questions for Candice

I don't have time off for myself and I feel too busy to be well. What holistic practices fit into a daily routine?

HI SIS! Life is crazy. WILD. But if you're busy, yet still have a few 'free' minutes – to chatter with Jesus or read your Bible – you're not self-indulgent or selfish. You're God-honoring and your spirit's being better nourished. It's not selfish, not at all, to care for your wellness. It's worship.

There have been other wellness things I've tried but have not stayed. I started this and fell off. How can I stay on?

Girl, I feel you too. Between the ups and downs of life, these are just reminders of what you've achieved so far. Understand this: with God on your side, you can do it. Pray over your goals, then make it your prayer to break down the steps into something you can handle. Picture each one of these as small wins, so that you can continue to trust that God still has your back as you achieve the rest with the strength you might not have had, before releasing it to His power. Add to that list of every brother and sister in Him alongside you — we're with you, too.

I'm hearing more and more about holistic wellness, but I'm not quite sure where to begin. Would you mind recommending some holistic practices for beginners?

Sweet sister, your path to whole health starts with letting go and letting God take your life's course. To do with it what He wills. To honor Him with how you treat your body. To nourish your body with food He blessed and allow it to move about according to His glory and pleasure. To pause during the day to praise Him for the blessing of breath and the opportunity to enjoy all that He has made. For the moments you take to manage wellness. Friends are another moment in a life waiting to be lived according to His purpose.

© 2024 - My Peace of Health, LLC

I'd like to pursue greater wellness but I can't afford the pricey products or services I've read/heard about. How can I stay within a budget and promote my well-being at the same time?

Trust me, girlfriend, God's blessings aren't determined by your budget. You don't have to spend a lot to keep yourself – get your creative juices flowing and find simple, inexpensive nutrition-packed meals. Walking is free! So is having company over. God's love is inexhaustible, your heart health is not!

I struggle with self-doubt and negative self-talk. How can I cultivate a more positive mindset and overcome these mental barriers?

Okay, let's get those lies out of there right now, because of Christ's grace, you can believe in who you are, so that when something comes into your mind that says, 'You're a failure, then you can read some Scriptures and say, I know God loves you, and I know He sent you here today to do such and such a thing. And you have your squad (and counselors) you can lean on. Stand up sister, you are fearfully and wonderfully made in His image.

© 2024 - My Peace of Health, LLC

© 2024 - My Peace of Health, LLC

© 2024 - My Peace of Health, LLC

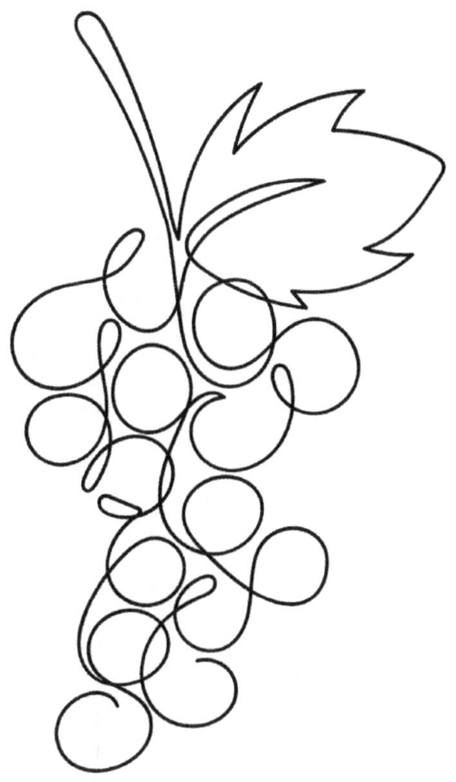

© 2024 - My Peace of Health, LLC

© 2024 - My Peace of Health, LLC

Introduction to the Easy On-the-Go Plant-Based Recipe Section

© 2024 - My Peace of Health, LLC

© 2024 - My Peace of Health, LLC

We are excited to present you with an easy on-the-go recipe collection of simple, plant-based lunches for busy people. Whether you have to rush off to a job, school, or just in between activities, we want to help with these quick, conscientious choices to make hectic days a little easier, plus a little more delicious and nutritious.

In our increasingly hurried world, 'easy' doesn't have to mean unhealthy or bland. By devoting just a little thought and effort to planning, plant-based cuisine can be wholesome, portable and convenient — and delicious, too.

Whether it's breakfast on the go, lunch to grab as you rush out the door, or a snack to fuel you throughout the day, every recipe is chosen to be quick and easy, as well as nutritious, made mostly with everyday ingredients and easy instructions, you will be preparing your meals and bites in no time, at home or on-the-go.

After all, when you eat poorly, you feel even more awful. Throughout this section, these nourishing, easy on-the-go plant-based recipes will show you a whole new world of what to eat while on the go. Just think no more greasy take-out or bland diet foods! Instead, think about snacking on raw food bars while commuting to work: feasting on fresh, raw veggies with vinaigrette while shopping or running errands; and dining on a fast and filling salad topped with a tasty dressing while traveling on the road.

© 2024 - My Peace of Health, LLC

© 2024 - My Peace of Health, LLC

Plant-Based Family Friendly Breakfast

© 2024 - My Peace of Health, LLC

© 2024 - My Peace of Health, LLC

Banana Oat Pancakes

Ingredients:

2 ripe bananas

1 cup rolled oats

1/2 cup plant-based milk (such as almond milk or oat milk)

1 teaspoon vanilla extract

1 teaspoon baking powder

Pinch of salt

Optional toppings: fresh berries, sliced bananas, maple syrup, or nut butter

Instructions:

In a blender or food processor, combine the ripe bananas, rolled oats, plant-based milk, vanilla extract, baking powder, and salt. Blend until smooth.

Heat a non-stick skillet or griddle over medium heat. Pour the pancake batter onto the skillet to form pancakes of your desired size.

Cook for 2-3 minutes on each side, or until golden brown and cooked through.

Serve the pancakes warm with your favorite toppings, such as fresh berries, sliced bananas, maple syrup, or nut butter.

© 2024 - My Peace of Health, LLC

Tofu Scramble

Ingredients:

1 block of firm tofu, drained and crumbled

1 tablespoon olive oil

1/2 onion, diced

1 bell pepper, diced

1 cup spinach or kale, chopped

2 cloves garlic, minced

1 teaspoon turmeric

Salt and pepper to taste

Optional toppings: avocado slices, salsa, nutritional yeast, or fresh herbs

Instructions:

Heat olive oil in a skillet over medium heat. Add diced onion and bell pepper, and sauté until softened about 5 minutes.

Add minced garlic and chopped spinach or kale to the skillet, and cook until the greens are wilted.

Add crumbled tofu to the skillet, along with turmeric, salt, and pepper. Stir well to combine and cook for another 5-7 minutes, or until the tofu is heated through and lightly browned.

Serve the tofu scramble hot, with optional toppings such as avocado slices, salsa, nutritional yeast, or fresh herbs.

© 2024 - My Peace of Health, LLC

Mixed Berry Smoothie Bowl

Ingredients:

2 ripe bananas, frozen

1 cup mixed berries (such as strawberries, blueberries, and raspberries), frozen

1/2 cup plant-based milk (such as almond milk or coconut milk)

Toppings: granola, sliced fresh fruit, shredded coconut, chia seeds, or hemp seeds

Instructions:

In a blender, combine the frozen bananas, mixed berries, and plant-based milk. Blend until smooth and creamy.

Pour the smoothie into bowls.

Top the smoothie bowls with your favorite toppings, such as granola, sliced fresh fruit, shredded coconut, chia seeds, or hemp seeds.

Serve immediately and enjoy!

© 2024 - My Peace of Health, LLC

<h1 style="text-align:center">Avocado Toast with Chickpea Smash</h1>

Ingredients:

2 ripe avocados

1 can (15 oz) chickpeas, drained and rinsed

1 tablespoon lemon juice

1 tablespoon olive oil

Salt and pepper to taste

4 slices of whole grain bread, toasted

Optional toppings: cherry tomatoes, sliced radishes, microgreens, or red pepper flakes

Instructions:

In a mixing bowl, mash the ripe avocados with a fork until smooth.

In a separate bowl, mash the chickpeas with a fork or potato masher until slightly chunky.

Combine the mashed avocados and mashed chickpeas in a bowl. Add lemon juice, olive oil, salt, and pepper, and mix well.

Spread the avocado-chickpea smash onto the toasted whole grain bread slices.

Top with your favorite toppings, such as cherry tomatoes, sliced radishes, microgreens, or red pepper flakes.

Serve immediately and enjoy!

© 2024 - My Peace of Health, LLC

Overnight Chia Seed Pudding

Ingredients:

1/4 cup chia seeds

1 cup plant-based milk (such as almond milk or coconut milk)

1 tablespoon maple syrup or agave nectar (optional)

1/2 teaspoon vanilla extract

Toppings: fresh fruit, nuts, seeds, or shredded coconut

Instructions:

In a mason jar or airtight container, combine chia seeds, plant-based milk, maple syrup or agave nectar (if using), and vanilla extract. Stir well to combine.

Cover the jar/container and refrigerate overnight, or for at least 4 hours, to allow the chia seeds to thicken and set.

Before serving, give the chia seed pudding a good stir. If it's too thick, you can add a splash of plant-based milk to reach your desired consistency.

Top the chia seed pudding with your favorite toppings, such as fresh fruit, nuts, seeds, or shredded coconut.

Serve chilled and enjoy!

© 2024 - My Peace of Health, LLC

Vegan Breakfast Burritos

Ingredients:

4 large flour tortillas (or whole grain tortillas)

 block of firm tofu, drained and crumbled

1 tablespoon olive oil

1 bell pepper, diced

1/2 onion, diced

1 cup black beans, cooked and drained

1 teaspoon ground cumin

Salt and pepper to taste

Optional toppings: avocado slices, salsa, chopped cilantro, or hot sauce

Instructions:

Heat olive oil in a skillet over medium heat. Add diced onion and bell pepper, and sauté until softened, about 5 minutes.

Add crumbled tofu to the skillet, along with ground cumin, salt, and pepper. Cook for 5-7 minutes, or until the tofu is heated through and lightly browned.

Warm the flour tortillas in a separate skillet or microwave.

Assemble the breakfast burritos by placing a scoop of the tofu scramble and black beans onto each tortilla. Add optional toppings such as avocado slices, salsa, chopped cilantro, or hot sauce.

© 2024 - My Peace of Health, LLC

Fold the sides of the tortilla over the filling, then roll it up tightly into a burrito.

Serve the vegan breakfast burritos warm and enjoy!

© 2024 - My Peace of Health, LLC

Coconut Chia Seed Breakfast Bowl

Ingredients:

1/4 cup chia seeds

1 cup coconut milk (canned or carton)

1 tablespoon maple syrup or agave nectar

1/2 teaspoon vanilla extract

Toppings: sliced banana, toasted coconut flakes, chopped nuts, or hemp seeds

Instructions:

In a bowl, combine chia seeds, coconut milk, maple syrup or agave nectar, and vanilla extract. Stir well to combine.

Cover the bowl and refrigerate for at least 4 hours, or overnight, to allow the chia seeds to thicken and set.

Before serving, give the chia seed mixture a good stir. If it's too thick, you can add a splash of coconut milk to reach your desired consistency.

Top the coconut chia seed pudding with sliced banana, toasted coconut flakes, chopped nuts, or hemp seeds.

Serve chilled and enjoy!

© 2024 - My Peace of Health, LLC

© 2024 - My Peace of Health, LLC

© 2024 - My Peace of Health, LLC

On the Go Plant-Based Lunch Ideas

© 2024 - My Peace of Health, LLC

© 2024 - My Peace of Health, LLC

Mason Jar Salads

Choose your favorite salad ingredients, such as:

- Dressing: Olive oil and balsamic vinegar, tahini dressing, or lemon vinaigrette.
- Vegetables: Chopped cucumbers, bell peppers, cherry tomatoes, shredded carrots, or roasted vegetables.
- Grains/Legumes: Cooked quinoa, chickpeas, black beans, or lentils.
- Greens: Spinach, kale, arugula, or mixed greens.

Layer the ingredients in a mason jar starting with dressing at the bottom, followed by grains/legumes, hearty vegetables, and greens on top. Seal the jar and refrigerate until ready to eat. Shake the jar before serving to mix the ingredients and distribute the dressing.

Veggie Wraps

- Whole grain wraps
- Hummus or mashed avocado
- Sliced vegetables such as cucumbers, bell peppers, carrots, and leafy greens
- Optional: Sprouts, shredded cabbage, or grated vegan cheese

Spread hummus or mashed avocado on a whole-grain wrap. Layer with sliced vegetables and any optional ingredients. Roll up tightly, slice in half, and wrap in parchment paper or aluminum foil for easy transport.

© 2024 - My Peace of Health, LLC

Portable Pasta Salad

- Whole grain pasta, cooked according to package instructions
- Chopped vegetables such as cherry tomatoes, broccoli florets, bell peppers, and cucumber
- Cooked chickpeas or white beans
- Vinaigrette dressing (homemade or store-bought)
- Optional: Fresh herbs like basil or parsley, olives, or sun-dried tomatoes

Toss the cooked pasta with chopped vegetables and beans. Drizzle with vinaigrette dressing and toss to coat evenly. Divide into individual containers for a quick and satisfying lunch option.

Energy-Boosting Trail Mix:

- Almonds
- Walnuts
- Pumpkin seeds
- Sunflower seeds
- Dried cranberries
- Dark chocolate chips or carob chips

Mix together the nuts, seeds, and dried fruits in a resealable bag or container. Adjust quantities based on personal preference. Enjoy as a convenient and nutritious snack on the go.

© 2024 - My Peace of Health, LLC

<h2 style="text-align:center">Chia Seed Pudding Cups</h2>

- Chia seeds
- Plant-based milk (such as almond milk or coconut milk)
- Sweetener (such as maple syrup or agave nectar)
- Fresh fruit, nuts, or coconut flakes for topping

In a small portable container, mix chia seeds with plant-based milk and sweetener. Let the mixture thicken in the refrigerator overnight. In the morning, top with fresh fruit, nuts, or coconut flakes before enjoying.

Homemade Veggie Sushi Rolls

- Sushi rice
- Nori sheets
- Sliced vegetables such as cucumber, avocado, bell peppers, and carrots
- Tofu or marinated tempeh (optional)

Soy sauce, wasabi, and pickled ginger for serving

Spread sushi rice evenly on a nori sheet. Layer sliced vegetables and tofu or tempeh on top. Roll tightly and slice into bite-sized pieces. Pack in a bento box or reusable container along with soy sauce, wasabi, and pickled ginger.

© 2024 - My Peace of Health, LLC

DIY Bento Box

- Sliced fresh fruit
- Raw vegetables (carrot sticks, cucumber slices, cherry tomatoes) with hummus or guacamole
- Whole grain crackers or rice cakes
- Roasted chickpeas or edamame
- Mini sandwiches or wraps filled with hummus, sliced vegetables, and leafy greens

Pack the bento box with a variety of plant-based snacks and small dishes into separate compartments. Customize with your favorite ingredients and enjoy a convenient and nutritious meal on the go!

These recipes are versatile, delicious, and perfect for busy days when you need a nutritious meal that you can take with you wherever you go!

© 2024 - My Peace of Health, LLC

© 2024 - My Peace of Health, LLC

© 2024 - My Peace of Health, LLC

Family Friendly Plant-Based Dinner Recipes

© 2024 - My Peace of Health, LLC

© 2024 - My Peace of Health, LLC

Chickpea and Vegetable Curry

Ingredients:

1 can chickpeas, drained and rinsed

1 onion, diced

2 cloves garlic, minced

1 bell pepper, diced

1 zucchini, diced

1 can coconut milk

2 tablespoons curry powder

1 teaspoon ground turmeric

Salt and pepper to taste

Cooked rice or naan for serving

Instructions:

In a large skillet, sauté the onion and garlic until softened.

Add the bell pepper and zucchini, and cook until tender.

Stir in the chickpeas, coconut milk, curry powder, turmeric, salt, and pepper. Simmer for 10-15 minutes.

Serve the curry over cooked rice or with naan.

© 2024 - My Peace of Health, LLC

Vegan Lentil Shepherd's Pie

Ingredients:

2 cups cooked lentils

1 onion, diced

2 carrots, diced

1 cup peas

2 cloves garlic, minced

2 tablespoons tomato paste

1 cup vegetable broth

Mashed potatoes for topping

Instructions:

Preheat the oven to 375°F (190°C).

In a skillet, sauté the onion and garlic until softened.

Add the carrots and cook until tender. Stir in the peas, cooked lentils, tomato paste, and vegetable broth. Simmer for 5-10 minutes.

Transfer the lentil mixture to a baking dish and top with mashed potatoes.

Bake for 20-25 minutes, or until the mashed potatoes are golden brown.

© 2024 - My Peace of Health, LLC

Veggie Stir-Fry with Tofu

Ingredients:

1 block tofu, pressed and cubed

Assorted vegetables (such as bell peppers, broccoli, carrots, and snap peas)

2 cloves garlic, minced

2 tablespoons soy sauce

1 tablespoon maple syrup

Cooked rice or noodles for serving

Instructions:

In a large skillet, sauté the tofu until golden brown on all sides.

Add the minced garlic and cook for another minute.

Stir in the assorted vegetables and cook until tender.

Add the soy sauce and maple syrup, and toss to coat.

Serve the stir-fry over cooked rice or noodles.

© 2024 - My Peace of Health, LLC

Spaghetti with Vegan Bolognese Sauce

Ingredients:

8 oz spaghetti

1 onion, diced

2 cloves garlic, minced

1 carrot, grated

1 zucchini, grated

1 can crushed tomatoes

1 tablespoon tomato paste

1 teaspoon dried oregano

Salt and pepper to taste

Instructions:

Cook the spaghetti according to package instructions.

In a skillet, sauté the onion and garlic until softened.

Add the grated carrot and zucchini, and cook until tender.

Stir in the crushed tomatoes, tomato paste, dried oregano, salt, and
 pepper. Simmer for 10-15 minutes.

Serve the sauce over the cooked spaghetti.

© 2024 - My Peace of Health, LLC

Black Bean and Sweet Potato Quesadillas

Ingredients:

1 can black beans, drained and rinsed

1 large sweet potato, cooked and mashed

1 bell pepper, diced

1 cup corn kernels

1 teaspoon ground cumin

1/2 teaspoon chili powder

4 large whole wheat tortillas

Vegan cheese (optional)

Instructions:

In a bowl, mix together the black beans, mashed sweet potato, bell pepper, corn kernels, ground cumin, and chili powder.

Spread the mixture onto half of each tortilla, then fold the tortillas in half.

Cook the quesadillas in a skillet over medium heat until golden brown on both sides.

Slice the quesadillas into wedges and serve with your favorite salsa or guacamole.

© 2024 - My Peace of Health, LLC

Spinach Stuffed Bell Peppers

Ingredients:

4 bell peppers, halved and seeded

1 onion, diced

2 cloves garlic, minced

2 cups fresh spinach

1 cup cooked quinoa

1 teaspoon dried thyme

Salt and pepper to taste

Instructions:

Preheat the oven to 375°F (190°C).

In a skillet, sauté the onion and garlic until softened.

Cook until tender. Stir in the spinach and cook until wilted.

Remove from heat and stir in the cooked quinoa, dried thyme, salt, and pepper.

Spoon the quinoa mixture into the halved bell peppers and place them in a baking dish.

Cover the dish with foil and bake for 25-30 minutes, or until the peppers are tender.

© 2024 - My Peace of Health, LLC

Coconut Lentil Curry

Ingredients:

1 cup dry lentils

1 onion, diced

2 cloves garlic, minced

1 bell pepper, diced

1 zucchini, diced

1 can of coconut milk

2 tablespoons curry powder

1 teaspoon ground turmeric

Salt and pepper to taste

Instructions:

Cook the lentils according to package instructions.

In a large skillet, sauté the onion and garlic until softened.

Add the bell pepper and zucchini, and cook until tender.

Stir in the cooked lentils, coconut milk, curry powder, turmeric, salt, and pepper. Simmer for 10-15 minutes.

Serve the curry over cooked rice or with naan.

© 2024 - My Peace of Health, LLC

© 2024 - My Peace of Health, LLC

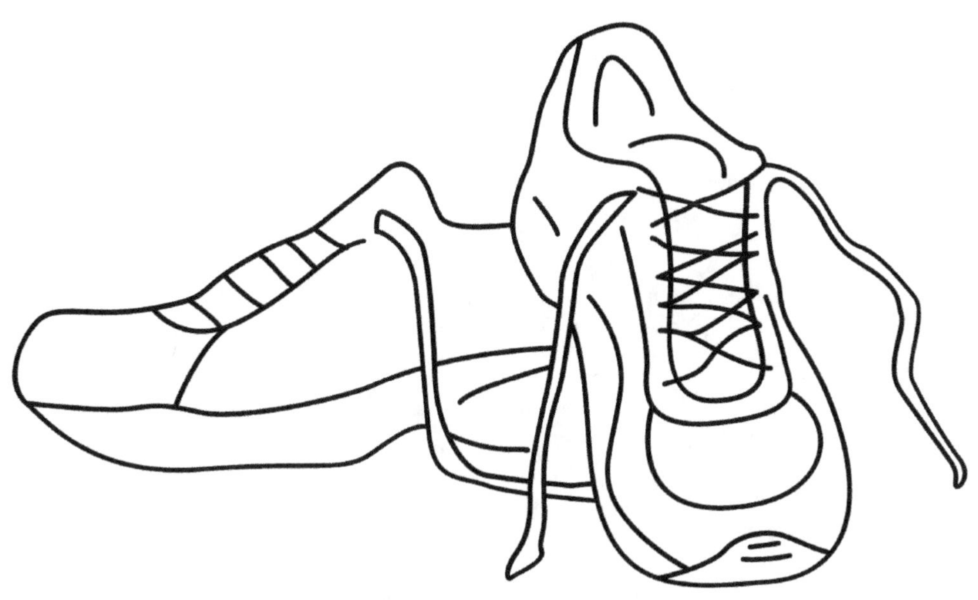

© 2024 - My Peace of Health, LLC

© 2024 - My Peace of Health, LLC

Women and Family Fitness Section

© 2024 - My Peace of Health, LLC

© 2024 - My Peace of Health, LLC

Welcome to our Women and Family Fitness Section! Our Women and Family Fitness Section is a dedicated space for women and families to explore how physical activity and exercise can help you and your family attain optimal health and wellness together. This program values women's unique needs and aims to bring joy back into your exercise life.

From prenatal and postnatal classes to workouts built for the female form to family-friendly programming, here you will find all of the women's health and fitness inspiration and services in one place.

However, to ensure your comfort and safety, and because your needs are unique to you, take some time before you delve into a plethora of workouts and activities to assess your health and fitness. What seems like a reasonable workout for one person – a walker among walkers, for example – may not be ideal for you. Therefore, before undertaking a new fitness program, especially if you have a known health issue or illness, consult a medical professional to make sure that what you are planning suits you and your current state of health.

Although exercise is good for most women, and families too, for cardiovascular health, strength, flexibility, and general happiness, it's important to tread the path of increased exercise cautiously, if you have any background medical conditions, injuries, or any other concerns.

With that said, let's embark on this journey together, prioritizing our health and well-being every step of the way.

© 2024 - My Peace of Health, LLC

© 2024 - My Peace of Health, LLC

Spiritual Strength: A Journey of Faith and Fitness for Christian Women

© 2024 - My Peace of Health, LLC

© 2024 - My Peace of Health, LLC

Week 1: Mindful Movement and Prayer

Day 1: Morning Walk and Prayer

Get up early every morning, go for a 20-minute walk outdoors, pray and talk to God, and think of three to five things that are blessing you, three to five things that are in your heart, and three to five things that you are thankful for.

Day 2: Pilates and Scripture Meditation

After a Pilates workout video (20 minutes) that concentrates on refining and lengthening the body, select from a passage of scripture and meditate on it at the same time.

Day 3: Stretching Routine and Worship

Perform a 20-minute stretching routine and remain as flexible as possible while also relaxing your mind and body. During this time, have some soothing worship music or hymns play in the background; you can also use the opportunity for prayer and praise.

Day 4: Dance and Devotion

Get your blood pumping and your unconscious inhibitions down with an unabashed 20-minute dance workout. Afterward, regular ritual items such as scripture reading or a Christian devotional invitation and a time of journaling your reflections.

Day 5: Restorative Stretching and Gratitude

Restorative, gentle stretching (20 minutes): go ahead and stretch out your body! Use light stretching to let go and help your body normalize. Give thanks to God for his love and the good things in your life (10 minutes): think of the blessings you have received and name them for yourself.

Day 6: Nature Walk and Reflection

© 2024 - My Peace of Health, LLC

Go for a half-hour walk in the natural world – in God's creation – let God's work and praise shape the words of your mouth as you quietly reflect, listen for and seek Him in His creation.

Day 7: Sabbath Rest

Set this day apart as a Holy Sabbath for rest, a day of worship and self-fulfillment, a blessing for you and all generations to come. Its purpose is to enable you to love God and become one with Him, sharing His holiness when you commit it to acts of prayer, reading, worship, or devotion, or to acts of kindness such as visiting the sick or welcoming the stranger.

Week 2: Strength and Surrender

Keep the format the same as Week 1; start with mindful movement, then follow with prayer and spiritual reflection, inviting God to deepen your union with him and to empower your body and spirit.

Week 3: Faith and Fitness Integration

Do some writing to integrate themes of faith and fitness, and reflect on how lessons from the gym or track may be applied to your spiritual life (e.g., how do you experience discipline, or perseverance, as you work out, and what role does trusting God play in your fitness?).

Week 4: Renewal and Rejuvenation

Think back over the previous three weeks, quiet your mind, renew your body, and Most importantly, renew your spirit. Reflect on where you feel marked today, in your life, and your relationship with God. Write down some intentions, positive declarations, goals, or aspirations.

As you experience these exercise programs, incorporate prayer, the reading and meditation of scriptures, and worship as central elements of your fitness ritual. As you exercise, listen to the voice of God for

© 2024 - My Peace of Health, LLC

guidance in co-creating the life you have always desired. Let the power of God sustain and equip you for life; his presence shall strengthen, comfort, and nourish you.

© 2024 - My Peace of Health, LLC

© 2024 - My Peace of Health, LLC

One Week of Family Fitness Activities

© 2024 - My Peace of Health, LLC

© 2024 - My Peace of Health, LLC

Day 1: Outdoor Adventure

- Morning: Family Nature Walk
  - Choose a scenic trail or park for a family nature walk.
  - Take time to appreciate God's creation and discuss the beauty of nature.
  - Encourage gratitude and reflection on God's provision and care.
- Afternoon: Picnic and Play
  - Pack a picnic lunch and enjoy fellowship together in a nearby park.
  - Play outdoor games like tag, Frisbee, or soccer, thanking God for the joy of movement and play.
  - End with a prayer of thanks for the time spent together as a family.

Day 2: Indoor Fitness Fun

- Morning: Family Dance Party
  - Play Christian music and have a dance party in the living room, praising God through movement and music.
  - Encourage creativity and expression as each family member dances joyfully before the Lord.
  - Take breaks for scripture reading and prayer throughout the dance session.
- Afternoon: Scripture Memory Challenge
  - Create a fun game or activity to help the family memorize Bible verses related to health and wellness.
  - Use movement-based exercises like jumping jacks or squats to reinforce scripture memory.
  - End with a time of prayer, asking God to help each family member apply His Word to their lives.

Day 3: Active Games and Challenges

- Morning: Obstacle Course of Faith

© 2024 - My Peace of Health, LLC

- Set up a backyard obstacle course with challenges that reflect Christian values, such as helping others, perseverance, and faithfulness.
    - Incorporate activities like carrying a "burden" (e.g., a heavy object) to represent bearing one another's burdens, and navigating obstacles while trusting God's guidance.
    - Conclude with a prayer thanking God for His strength and guidance in overcoming obstacles.
- Afternoon: Scripture Scavenger Hunt
    - Create a scavenger hunt around the house or yard with clues that lead to Bible verses related to physical health and spiritual well-being.
    - As each clue is found, take time to read and discuss the corresponding scripture together as a family.
    - End with a prayer of gratitude for the wisdom and guidance found in God's Word.

Day 4: Sports and Recreation

- Morning: Family Sports Day
    - Participate in a variety of sports activities together, such as basketball, soccer, or volleyball, thanking God for the opportunity to use our bodies in physical activity.
    - Focus on teamwork, sportsmanship, and encouragement as you compete and play together.
    - Conclude with a prayer of thanks for the joy of fellowship and friendly competition.
- Afternoon: Creation Fitness Challenge
    - Create a fitness challenge inspired by God's creation, such as "Leap Like a Gazelle" or "Swim Like a Fish."
    - Incorporate exercises that mimic animal movements and behaviors while reflecting on God's creativity and design.
    - Conclude with a prayer of praise for the wonders of God's creation and the blessing of physical health.

© 2024 - My Peace of Health, LLC

Day 5: Mind-Body Connection

- Morning: Scripture Stretching Session
    - Lead the family in a stretching session while meditating on scripture verses related to strength, peace, and renewal.
    - Encourage each family member to reflect on the meaning of the verses as they stretch their bodies and minds.
    - Conclude with a prayer asking God to strengthen and renew our body, soul, and spirit.
- Afternoon: Family Prayer Walk
    - Take a prayer walk around the neighborhood or local park, praying for the needs of your family, community, and world.
    - Use nature as inspiration for prayer, thanking God for His provision and asking for His guidance and protection.
    - Conclude with a time of thanksgiving and praise for the opportunity to connect with God and one another through prayer.

Day 6: DIY Fitness Circuit

- Morning: Family Fitness Circuit
    - Set up a circuit of fitness stations in the backyard or living room, each with a different exercise or activity.
    - Incorporate scripture verses at each station to encourage spiritual reflection and motivation.
    - Conclude with a prayer of thanks for the strength and endurance God provides as we care for our bodies.
- Afternoon: Fruit of the Spirit Workout
    - Create a workout routine based on the fruits of the Spirit (love, joy, peace, patience, kindness, goodness, faithfulness, gentleness, and self-control).
    - Assign each fruit of the Spirit to a specific exercise or movement, reflecting on how it relates to physical fitness and spiritual growth.
    - Conclude with a prayer asking God to cultivate His fruit in our lives as we seek to honor Him in all we do.

© 2024 - My Peace of Health, LLC

Day 7: Rest and Reflection

- Morning: Sabbath Rest
    - Take a day of rest and reflection, honoring the Sabbath as a time of physical, emotional, and spiritual renewal.
    - Spend time in prayer, scripture reading, and worship as a family, thanking God for His faithfulness and provision.
    - Reflect on the week's activities and blessings, expressing gratitude for the opportunity to grow closer to God and one another.
- Afternoon: Family Devotional Time
    - Gather together for a family devotional time, reading scripture, singing hymns, and sharing testimonies of God's goodness and grace.
    - Take turns praying for one another's needs and concerns, lifting each other up in faith and encouragement.
    - End with a time of fellowship and celebration, rejoicing in the love and fellowship of the family of God.

© 2024 - My Peace of Health, LLC

© 2024 - My Peace of Health, LLC

© 2024 - My Peace of Health, LLC

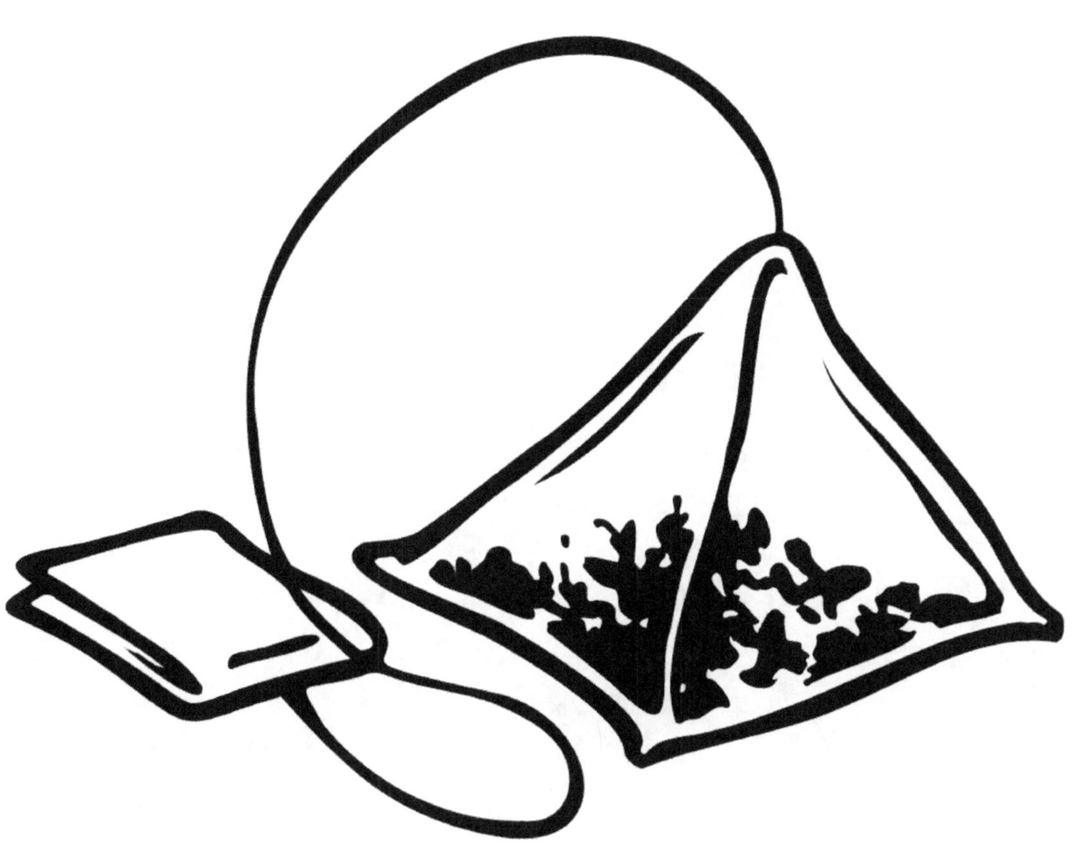

© 2024 - My Peace of Health, LLC

More Wellness Resources

© 2024 - My Peace of Health, LLC

© 2024 - My Peace of Health, LLC

Serenity Aromatherapy Room Spray:

Ingredients:

- 10 drops of lavender essential oil
- 5 drops of bergamot essential oil
- 1 cup distilled water

Instructions:

1. Mix the essential oils with distilled water in a spray bottle.
2. Shake well before each use and spray in the air or on linens.
3. Lavender and bergamot are both soothing scents that can promote relaxation and peace.

Peaceful Bath Soak:

Ingredients:

- 1 cup Epsom salt
- 1/2 cup baking soda
- 10 drops of chamomile essential oil
- 5 drops of cedarwood essential oil.

Instructions:

1. Mix Epsom salt and baking soda in a bowl, then add the essential oils and mix well.
2. Add the mixture to a warm bath and soak for at least 20 minutes.
3. This bath soak can help relax muscles and calm the mind.

© 2024 - My Peace of Health, LLC

Calming Lavender Chamomile Pillow Mist:

Ingredients:

- 1/2 cup distilled water
- 1 tablespoon witch hazel
- 10 drops of lavender essential oil
- 10 drops of chamomile essential oil.

Instructions:

1. Mix all ingredients in a spray bottle and shake well before each use.
2. Spray lightly onto pillows and bedding before sleep to create a calming atmosphere and promote restful sleep.

Tranquility Massage Oil:

Ingredients:

- 1/4 cup sweet almond oil
- 5 drops ylang-ylang essential oil
- 5 drops patchouli essential oil
- 3 drops of clary sage essential oil.

Instructions:

1. Mix all ingredients in a small bottle and shake well before each use.
2. Use this massage oil to soothe tired muscles and calm the mind during self-massage or partner massages.

© 2024 - My Peace of Health, LLC

© 2024 - My Peace of Health, LLC

© 2024 - My Peace of Health, LLC

Holistic Women's Coaching and Holistic Family Coaching

We hope that as you take time to read 'My Peace of Health' you will join our family in a holistic wellness and faith-centered living experience. body, mind, and spirit. Welcome to our family! Come with us as we embrace holistic wellness and faith-centered living. It's time to discover what it means to be 'One!'

At the core of our programs is our motivation to help you heal from the inside out: to rebuild your body, find emotional stability, reconnect with God, and get back in sync with your family.

Embrace Holistic Wellness

Our Women's Holistic Coaching Program is a sacred space to cultivate your holistic well-being from a Christian worldview centered around prayerful reflection and scripture study, as well as practical coaching to help you better understand how God wants you to:
• care for your body
• eat well
• cultivate inner peace and greater resilience.

Nurture Your Family's Well-Being

Through interactive sessions and age-appropriate activities in our Family Holistic Coaching Program, we invite families to spend quality time together nourishing their bodies as the divine temples they are, improving their emotional resilience and bond, and enhancing their spiritual connection.

Experience Transformation

Together At 'My Peace of Health', we believe that true transformation takes place within the community. That is why we don't just provide facts and resources, but a community for healing where you can be accompanied by people on the same path that you are on.

© 2024 - My Peace of Health, LLC

Start Your Journey Today

Are you ready to experience the peace, joy, and abundance that come from living in alignment with God's plan for your life? Join us at "My Peace of Health" and embark on a journey of holistic wellness and spiritual growth for you and your family. Together, let's discover the transformative power of faith-centered living.

Visit mypeaceofhealth.com to learn more and start your journey today.

© 2024 - My Peace of Health, LLC

Resources for Health and Wellness

Books:
- *The Ministry of Healing* by E.G. White: A profound exploration of holistic health from a spiritual perspective.
- *Counsels on Diet and Foods* by E.G. White: Practical advice on nutrition and healthy eating habits.
- *Depression: The Way Out* and *Proof Positive* by Neil Nedley: Comprehensive guides to understanding and managing mental health through lifestyle changes.
- *OVERCOMING AUTOIMMUNITY: One Physician's Step by Step Journey to Victory Over Her Chronic Illnesses* by Karla Montague-Brown MD: A personal account of triumph over chronic illnesses, offering insights and strategies for overcoming autoimmune conditions.

Websites:
- AdventHealth: A comprehensive online platform offering articles, resources, and programs designed to promote physical, mental, and spiritual well-being.
- Adventist Health Ministries: A hub for health-related resources, including tips, articles, and programs supporting a holistic approach to wellness.
- NewStart: A dedicated resource providing holistic lifestyle medicine guidance, including the N.E.W.S.T.A.R.T. principles, for individuals and communities seeking transformative health changes.
- Crowntosolewellness.com: Offers coaching and resources for overcoming autoimmunity, guided by the expertise of Karla Montague-Brown MD

© 2024 - My Peace of Health, LLC

© 2024 - My Peace of Health, LLC

About the Author

Candice Leanos is a passionate advocate for holistic wellness: besides being a Christian Holistic Wellness Coach, Candice is also a wife and homeschooling mother of five children. She has a unique story about her path to holistic wellness. Candice has always been committed to education and experience as well as faith.

With numerous certifications in Family Ministries Leadership, Plant-Based Nutrition, Fitness Instruction, and more, Candice is dedicated to journeying alongside her clients as they create life transformations that lead to increased joy and spiritual growth.

My Peace of Health LLC, which she founded and leads as CEO, is the embodiment of the principles that she teaches in her book My Peace of Health. Her book provides practical health knowledge and spiritual wisdom for achieving optimal health.

Her background in Practical Nursing and her passion for the holistic way of life guide her to emphasize the importance of a balanced approach to wellness. In everything she does – from coaching to speaking engagements to writing – Candice continues to share her vision of life lived to its fullest, a life that is abundant, energetic, and serene.

© 2024 - My Peace of Health, LLC

© 2024 - My Peace of Health, LLC

Credits:

- Research published in the American Journal of Clinical Nutrition
- Dr. Michael Greger, author of How Not to Die
- American Heart Association
- Dweck, C. S. (2006). Mindset: The New Psychology of Success. Random House.
- Brown, B. (2012). Daring Greatly: How the Courage to Be Vulnerable Transforms the Way We Live, Love, Parent, and Lead. Penguin Random House.
- Siegel, D. J. (2010). Mindsight: The New Science of Personal Transformation. Bantam.
- Nedley, N., Derose, D., & Scharffenberg, J. A. (1999). *Proof Positive: How to Reliably Combat Disease and Achieve Optimal Health Through Nutrition and Lifestyle.* Hardcover, Publisher: Nedley Publishing.

Bibliography

- Rudolph, Wilma. *Wilma Rudolph: Against All Odds.* New York: Putnam, 1999.

© 2024 - My Peace of Health, LLC

© 2024 - My Peace of Health, LLC

www.ingramcontent.com/pod-product-compliance
Lightning Source LLC
Chambersburg PA
CBHW081209260726

48653CB00010BA/3577